There Is a Choice: Homeoprophylaxis

Cilla Whatcott, PhD, HD RHom, CCH

Copyright © 2014 Cilla Whatcott
All rights reserved.
ISBN-13: 978-1502460257

Because of the dynamic nature of the internet, any web addresses or links contained in this book may have changed since publication and may no longer be valid.
Stock images are from istockphoto.com. Personal photographs taken by Cilla or family and friends of Cilla Whatcott.

Thanks to Richard Nunez and Sarah Perman for the cover design.

To all those who have questioned
and to all those who seek more
answers for the benefit of children everywhere.

CONTENTS

	Acknowledgments	i
	Forward	3
1	In the Beginning	7
2	Big Business of Vaccines	13
3	Immunity	25
4	Vaccine Studies	37
5	Homeoprophylaxis	49
6	Historical Evidence	63
7	Current Evidence of HP	75
8	Dr. Isaac Golden	81
9	Making Choices	89
10	Your Legal Rights	95
11	Applying Homeoprophylaxis	101
12	CEASE Therapy	115
13	Conclusion	121

ACKNOWLEDGMENTS

To my children who have taught me more than I ever imagined possible.

To Neal, who has provided a lifetime of love and safety
in which to learn and grow.

To all those children who depend on the love and wisdom
of parents in order to thrive.

And to Isaac – thank you for living your dharma.

Also by Cilla Whatcott
(Co-authored by Kate Birch)

The Solution - Homeoprophylaxis: The Vaccine Alternative

FOREWORD

There is a reality to Cilla Whatcott's book, *There Is A Choice,* that is often missing in purely academic texts, and it comes from her recounting of a very personal and deeply felt story involving her experience with raising her own children and the challenges involved with the decision whether to vaccinate or not.

Most parents do not discuss whether to vaccinate. They accept orthodox advice, and often see and hear negative descriptions of parents who choose not to vaccinate by the media and from doctors and politicians. UNLESS, of course, they experience vaccine damage first-hand, or hear of or see the experiences of trusted friends or relatives with vaccine-damaged children.

And so some concerned parents choose to start researching the safety and effectiveness of routine vaccination, and the first thing they find is that they have not been told the full story. It is very possible that their local doctor or nurse also does not know the full story, because it is not taught during University courses and there is a disincentive for health professionals to look beyond the conventional wisdom of pharmaceutical medicine.

But this discovery breeds distrust in directives from health authorities. After all when you find that a previously trusted authority has not been completely honest about one thing then the next question becomes – what else have they failed to tell me?

Then some parents choose to stop vaccinating their children because of evidence-based concerns about the possible dangers to the intellectual, emotional and physical health of their children. But that is a less than perfect solution because some (not all) of the vaccine-preventable disease are potentially very damaging, and they feel exposed and vulnerable – and they are told "how would you feel if your child is harmed by a potentially preventable disease?"

And it is here that Cilla's book becomes an invaluable resource, showing these parents that there are more than two choices: vaccinate or don't vaccinate. In fact, there is a middle way where their child can be significantly protected against the most potentially serious diseases without any risk of toxic damage.

Homeoprophylaxis (HP) is controversial with a minority of homeopaths, let alone with the Big Pharma establishment. However Cilla shows that HP was first used by the founder of homeopathy over 200 years ago, and is currently used by government health departments around the world with millions of people.

It is a complex topic which Cilla makes approachable for parents, with simple and clear explanations of the evidence available, interspersed with her own experiences as a parent.

And parents find that they do have choices when it comes to safely preventing potentially serious infectious diseases in their children, or in themselves because HP can be used for people of any age and for any infectious disease.

This is a subject where misinformation and fear are often used as weapons to coerce parents to behave in a particular way, and to hand over responsibility for the care of their children to individuals and institutions who have little interest in the wellbeing of the children, only for corporate profits and personal and professional status.

But truth is the most effective antidote to fear. The truths given by Cilla – however inconvenient to some – have the real potential to give needed support to troubled parents, and give them options which will help them provide their children with a better opportunity for lifelong health.

Finally, this is not a book advising parents that they should not vaccinate their children. The best a parent can do is to collect reliable evidence and make the most informed decision possible. Then they can live with their decision because they know they have done their best. But to do this they need honest and objective evidence. And this is where Cilla's book becomes invaluable – in providing reliable evidence to assist parents in making informed choices.

Isaac Golden, PhD, DHom, ND, BEc (Hon)
2014

1 IN THE BEGINNING

In most ways I'm just like you. I care deeply about my children and have struggled to make the right choices in raising them. We spend so many years protecting them, teaching them, guiding them, and keeping them safe from all the real and imagined dangers that lie in wait. Regardless of our careers or interests or occupations, they are always in the forefront of our minds and hearts as we pick and choose what to feed them, what to teach them, what to protect them from, or expose them to.

I remember looking away for a moment as we were at the desk, checking into a hotel in Honolulu. I turned and Max was gone! He was 18 months old and in gear with no brakes most of the time. Why hadn't I held his hand? How could I be so careless, so self-centered as to be weary of keeping constant vigilance and looking away? This was 1989 and the world was a safer place than it is now, but I still envisioned every possible horror imaginable during the three minutes before we found him! He was a mere 40 feet away, calmly sitting on the floor, mesmerized by the revolving door.

That was my first experience of how one can age very rapidly from fright, worry, and regret over having made a poor decision.

The decisions never end. There's walking – leading to the risk of losing them in public places. There's food – will I nourish them properly? Should I stand my ground or allow their "natural intelligence" to choose what their body needs? There's clothing – one of the lesser wars unless like mine they have very particular tastes regarding fit, feel and features of every item of apparel. There's school – this can constitute lots of sleep loss considering the monumental impact that educational philosophies, friends, teachers and school lunches can have. And then of course, there is whether or not to vaccinate.

This one never factored into my worries. After all, we were taught that vaccines protect from deadly diseases. Vaccines have been around for a long time. Vaccines have been tested and proven safe. So I dutifully marched my two little boys into the pediatrician's office and steeled myself against the flailing and shrieking long enough to allow the nurse to get in the jabs. I cuddled them as we left, soothing their indignation, sometimes stopping for ice cream on the way home to reward us all for making the right choice. Why would I even question such a decision? And I didn't, until Lily came along.

Lily was my third child. She was the game changer. Who would have guessed that this tiny baby could be such a powerful force for transformation? But then again, I think I can say that each one of my kids had that power and have made me who I am today. A very different person than I was B.C. (before children).

Lily was born in China, in the city of Jiujang, in Jiangxhi Province. She was eleven months old when we traveled to get her. We were no strangers to adoption. Max was eight years old at the time and we had adopted him from Taipei, Taiwan when he was just four months old. In between Max and Lily, I gave birth to Gus. This was quite the miraculous event as I had only one operational fallopian tube and it was declared blocked after lengthy and invasive testing, so I had settled into the realization that if I wanted a family, it would be through adoption.

We knew the drill. Many months of validating who you are, that you are healthy, financially stable, mentally sound, legally clean and have the patience of Job to wade through paperwork, certifications and the tedious wait for THE phone call.

We were a tad smug in our parenting expertise since we had two healthy boys at home who had obviously survived all our beginning parenting skills, inconsistent feeding schedules and lackadaisical bedtime routines. And after the hotel lobby escapade, I was very diligent in never taking my eyes off Max in public when he zoomed into high speed. We were well "experienced."

Lily was beautiful. What baby girl wouldn't be as the encore to two little boys? She only weighed ten pounds and could barely hold up her head. Her tiny features were so delicate and she was as quiet as a mouse. She didn't cry at all and slept through the night without a peep. She was perfect. We gave away the umbrella stroller we brought with us to China and instead bought a few yards of cotton cloth, which we tied in a knot and draped over my husband's shoulders to create an impromptu sling. She snuggled inside as content as a baby roo. The three of us were in heaven.

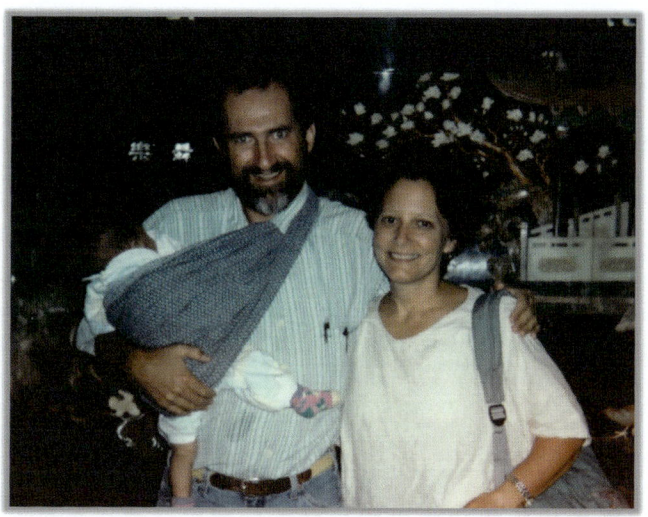

The flight home was long. We were living in the Marshall Islands at the time so took flights to Hong Kong, then Honolulu and then home. We wanted to return as quickly as possible to introduce Lily to her brothers. She was fussy on the flight and we assumed a possible ear infection might be brewing.

Once home we took her to the pediatrician to check her ears. She confirmed that they were a bit red and then suggested that she needed her appropriate vaccines. Having never even questioned vaccines, I agreed and Lily was given her DPT, hepatitis B, polio, and I believe the MMR. What I know now is that this amounts to eight separate disease agents at once, not to mention the additives in each injection. A chemical cocktail.

Looking back, I can see that Lily was suffering from "failure to thrive," or the lack of weight gain and physical growth that children suffer when inadequately nurtured and underfed. Combine this with a developing immune system and the trauma of leaving the familiarity of the orphanage, and you have a child who was very vulnerable.

Shortly after her vaccines, Lily's leg swelled to twice the size. Within a few hours she became more and more agitated and began to cry loudly. Long woeful shrieks were coming from her and nothing soothed her.

I took her temperature and it was 103 F. and rising. She was clearly in great distress and I ran her back to the pediatrician where she was diagnosed with aseptic meningitis. This is an inflammation of the membrane covering the brain and spinal cord. She was given IV antibiotics and her fever continued to climb to about 105 degrees F.

I tried to accept the fact that she might die and spent the next forty eight hours holding her warm, limp body and praying.

This was in 1996 and living in the Marshall Islands, the World Wide Web was not yet a common addition to every home. I did have a Merck Manual though. The Merck Manual is one of the world's most trusted medical references. First published in 1899, The "Merck Manual of Diagnosis and Therapy" is a concise and complete medical reference for doctors, medical students, and healthcare professionals. I love non-fiction. This was just one of the tomes I owned for recreational reading.

From its pages I read: *"Disorders and drugs are common causes of meningitis. Disorders that most commonly cause meningitis include disorders that cause inflammation, including the inflammation that occurs when the body's immune system malfunctions and attacks the body's own tissues (autoimmune disorders)."* [i1] The culpable drugs listed included, you guessed it, vaccines.

Eager for validation, back I went to the pediatrician, armed with my information and certain she would be proud of me for unearthing the actual cause of Lily's illness. I was sadly mistaken.

She informed me with complete confidence and authority that there was no connection whatsoever to the vaccines. Completely impossible. And furthermore, she delivered a terse lecture on the horrors of children dying from communicable diseases and how she had seen these horrors in the field. End of conversation.

I was speechless.

---

[1] Beer MH, Porter RS, Jones TV (2006 18th Edition). The Merck Manual of Diagnosis and Therapy. Hoboken, NJ: Wiley, John & Sons, Incorporated.

In the months and years that followed, I underwent a total reorganization of my belief system. There are some things we hold sacred. My respect for the medical profession used to be one of them.

Where do we turn when our kids are sick or suffering? Who do we ask about feeding schedules, naps, thumb sucking and nutrition? Their doctor, of course!

The stark realization hit me with full force that no one was going to look out for my kids as I do. It was up to me. Period. Others were motivated by saving face, dogma, pride, or even just putting in their eight hour work day. My children were my twenty four hour responsibility. They were the love of my life and they depended upon me to be there, know what to do and do it right.

The sheer responsibility felt overwhelming. But at the same time, it felt somehow empowering. I wasn't going to trust what someone else told me without doing my own research ever again. I was done being a conventional medicine groupie.

We left the Marshall Islands three years later in 1999. We had been there for ten years. It was paradise on earth. No cars, no crime, perfect weather near the equator and azure blue water. I took the kids swimming in the bathtub-like, warm lagoon, fringed by a pristine vacant beach. It felt like our own private sand box and kiddie pool. The boys raced crabs and collected coconuts. We knew almost everyone on the island and the school, the store and hospital were all staffed with expatriates like ourselves – people of every race and creed who contracted to companies like GE, Lockheed, or Massachusetts Institute of Technology. It felt like a summer camp filled with family and friends. We left there in 1999 and returned to the U.S. with mixed emotions.

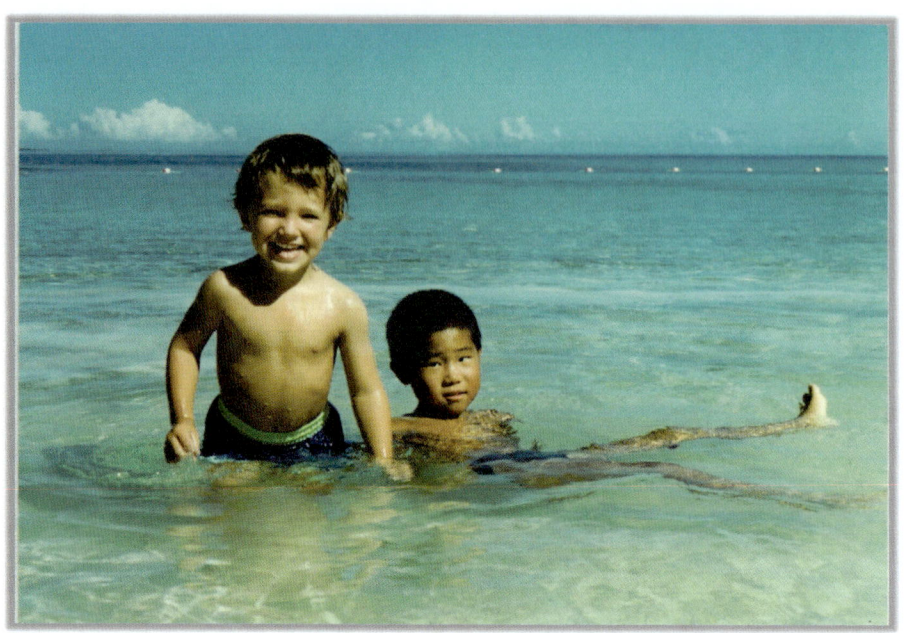

Gus and Max in Kwajalein Lagoon at Emon Beach

2 BIG BUSINESS OF VACCINES

The world had changed since 1989 when we left the U.S. One of the most noticeable changes was the addition of direct marketing of pharmaceutical drugs on television. It seemed almost ludicrous to hear the long list of possible side effects rattled off at the end of each ad. The boys would sit mesmerized as they listened and then burst into laughter as they tried to recite all the bizarre possibilities. "…headaches, muscle spasms rashes, diarrhea, gas, and possible death." Even preteens could see the senselessness of taking a drug that could result in something even worse than what you originally had.

Shortly before we had returned stateside, both the hepatitis B and varicella vaccine had been added to the recommended list of childhood immunizations. I found this curious since chicken pox is a relatively benign disease and as I later learned, instrumental in maturing the immune system. My entire family had had chickenpox and were none the worse as a result. And the chances of hepatitis B being contracted by an infant seemed ridiculously low since this disease is transmitted sexually or by shared blood products. I then did some reading and here's what I learned.

In 1995 The Center for Disease Control and Prevention (CDC) designed a surveillance study to determine the medical effects of the varicella vaccine in three separate communities: Antelope Valley, California; West Philadelphia, Pennsylvania; and Travis County, Texas. This was titled Varicella Active Surveillance Project, or VASP. [2] Antelope Valley was an especially ideal location as it was an isolated area of about 300,000 residents who rarely sought healthcare outside of the community. As a result, changes over time could be accurately monitored.

One of the researchers, Gary Goldman, PhD, found something very disturbing. Second guessing himself, he combed through the medical literature to see if anything similar existed. What he found was this:

From the United Kingdom in 1992, two university researchers examined the epidemiological implications of world-wide varicella vaccination and made this summary:
> "Under some conditions, mass application of such vaccines may have the impact of increasing herpes zoster (shingles) incidence. The results presented here indicate that before starting any vaccination programme against varicella, its consequences need to be assessed in much more depth." [3]

And then in 1996 University of Oxford researchers concluded:
> "There is a danger of increased herpes zoster incidence following reduction in varicella incidence if subclinical infections play a part in assisting the immune system in keeping the latent virus in check. It would be wise for health authorities introducing the widespread use of varicella vaccine in healthy children to monitor epidemiology of herpes zoster both before and after the introduction of vaccination for early signs in the increase of herpes zoster. If varicella vaccination was to increase the incidence of herpes zoster then this change in morbidity would probably outweigh the benefits of reduced incidence of chickenpox." [4]

The repeated exposure to wild varicella through contact with children or grandchildren provides what is known as an "exogenous boost" to the immune system. This activates cell mediated immunity and protects from shingles. Trying to eliminate naturally occurring chickenpox could result in increased cases of shingles, a much more

---

[2] 2014. Retrieved from: http://www.ncbi.nlm.nih.gov/pubmed/22659447

[3] Garnett GP, Grenfell BT. The epidemiology of varicella-zoster virus infections: the influence of varicella on the prevalence of herpes zoster. Epidemiol. Infect. 1992 Jun; 108(3):513-528.

[4] Ferguson NM, Anderson RM, Garnett GP. Mass vaccination to control chickenpox: the influence of zoster. Proc. Natl. Acad. Sci. U.S.A., 1996 Jul. 9;93(14):7231-7235.

painful and potentially life threatening disease. [5]

This is what Dr. Goldman was actually seeing. Antelope Valley's shingles rate was higher than any expected norm. Furthermore, he was witnessing that children ten years old and younger were now presenting with shingles at the same rate as adults over the age of forty. This was previously unheard of! The incidence of shingles has always increased with each decade of life after the age of forty, presumably due to the decrease in exogenous boosts as the elderly have less and less contact with children having wild chickenpox.

It seems that Mother Nature knew what she was doing when she created chickenpox as a benign childhood disease. Tipping this balance has wreaked havoc with the natural order and resulted in more adults suffering with shingles since the chickenpox vaccine was added to the recommended list in 1995.

Dr. Goldman's expectation was that his superiors from the CDC would be happy that he had discovered this in the surveillance. They were silent. They did not publish the papers he had written, nor did they heed his warnings regarding the possible intensification that would be seen with cases of shingles. His censored research was subsequently published in other peer-reviewed medical journals. [6]

---

[5] Thomas SL, Wheeler JG, Hall AJ. Contacts with varicella or with children and protection against herpes zoster in adults: a case–control study. Lancet 2002;360(9334):678–682.

[6] Goldman G. Varicella susceptibility and incidence of herpes zoster among children and adolescents in a community under active surveillance [Vaccine, 2003 Oct. 1;21 (27-30): 4238-4242]; Incidence of herpes zoster among children and adolescents in a community with moderate varicella vaccination coverage [Vaccine, 2003 Oct. 1;21(27-30):4243-4249]; Using capture-recapture methods to assess varicella incidence in a community under active surveillance[Vaccine, 2003 Oct 1;21(27-30):4250-4255]; Cost analysis of universal varicella vaccination in the U.S. taking into account the closely related herpes zoster epidemiology [Vaccine, 2005 May; 23(25):3349-3355]; Response to Letter to Editor by Jumaan: Goldman's role in the Varicella Active Surveillance Project [Vaccine 2004 Sep 3; 22(25-26):3232-3236]; Universal varicella vaccination: Efficacy trends and effect on herpes zoster [International Journal of Toxicology, 2005 July-Aug;24(4):205-213]; The Case Against Universal Varicella Vaccination [International Journal of Toxicology, 2006 Sep-Oct;25(5):313-317].

Many European countries did not adopt the recommendation for the vaccine.

Merck, one step ahead in the consumer market, created yet another vaccine called Zostavax. Zostavax is simply a larger-than-normal dose of Varivax, and is used in older adults to presumably protect against shingles. It was only tested in 50-59 year olds who were then monitored for 1.3 years post vaccination. In this cohort, for that amount of time, the vaccine was 70% effective. [7] The possible side effects are listed as: "Serious vaccine-related adverse reactions that have occurred following vaccination with ZOSTAVAX include asthma exacerbation and polymyalgia rheumatica. Other serious adverse events reported following vaccination with ZOSTAVAX include cardiovascular events (congestive heart failure, pulmonary edema)."[8]

Merck is enjoying healthy returns on this biologically assisted disease enhancement. Merck's third quarter earnings for 2013 totaled $11 million. If other quarters reflected similar profits, this would amount to $44 million dollars. [9]

More Deception

I've chosen to share just a few highlights of how pharmaceutical manufacturers have manipulated information to the benefit of their bottom line – profit. These illustrations are historically significant as they impacted, and continue to impact, the health outcomes of our children.

On Aug. 27, 2014 a senior scientist at the Centers for Disease Control publicly admitted[10] that he and other CDC officials, including the current CDC's Director of Immunization Safety,[11][12] published a study about MMR

[7] MerckVaccines.com 2014 retrieved from:
https://www.merckvaccines.com/Products/Zostavax/Pages/efficacy/ZEST

[8] MerckVaccines.com 2014 retrieved from:
https://www.merckvaccines.com/Products/Zostavax/Pages/efficacy/ZESTsafey

[9] http://www.mercknewsroom.com/news-release/corporate-news/merck-announces-third-quarter-2013-financial-results

[10] Thompson WW. Statement of William W. Thompson, PhD, Regarding the 2014 Article Examining the Possibility of a Relationship Between MMR Vaccine and Autism. Morgan Verkamp, LLC Aug. 27, 2014.

vaccine safety in 2004 [13] that "omitted statistically significant information" and "did not follow the final study protocol." His public statement is as follows:

> "My name is William Thompson. I am a Senior Scientist with the Centers for Disease Control and Prevention, where I have worked since 1998.
>
> I regret that my coauthors and I omitted statistically significant information in our 2004 article published in the journal Pediatrics. The omitted data suggested that African American males who received the MMR vaccine before age 36 months were at increased risk for autism. Decisions were made regarding which findings to report after the data were collected, and I believe that the final study protocol was not followed.
>
> I want to be absolutely clear that I believe vaccines have saved and continue to save countless lives. I would never suggest that any parent avoid vaccinating children of any race. Vaccines prevent serious diseases, and the risks associated with their administration are vastly outweighed by their individual and societal benefits.
>
> My concern has been the decision to omit relevant findings in a particular study for a particular sub group for a particular vaccine. There have always been recognized risks for vaccination and I believe it is the responsibility of the CDC to properly convey the risks associated with receipt of those vaccines.
>
> I have had many discussions with Dr. Brian Hooker over the last 10 months regarding studies the CDC has carried out regarding vaccines and neurodevelopmental outcomes including autism spectrum disorders. I share his belief that CDC decision-making

---

[11] DeStefano F. Articles by Frank DeStefano, MD. Pub Med Accessed Aug. 29, 2014.

[12] Attkisson S. (Audio) CDC Addresses Allegation on Vaccine-Autism Link Omission. Aug. 29, 2014.

[13] CDC. CDC Statement Regarding 2004 Pediatrics Article "Age at First Measles-Mumps-Rubella Vaccination in Children with Autism and School-matched Control Subjects: A Population Based Study in Metropolitan Atlanta." CDC.GOV Aug. 25, 2014.

and analyses should be transparent. I was not, however, aware that he was recording any of our conversations, nor was I given any choice regarding whether my name would be made public or my voice would be put on the Internet.

I am grateful for the many supportive e-mails that I have received over the last several days. I will not be answering further questions at this time. I am providing information to Congressman William Posey, and of course will continue to cooperate with Congress. I have also offered to assist with reanalysis of the study data or development of further studies. For the time being, however, I am focused on my job and my family.

Reasonable scientists can and do differ in their interpretation of information. I will do everything I can to assist any unbiased and objective scientists inside or outside the CDC to analyze data collected by the CDC or other public organizations for the purpose of understanding whether vaccines are associated with an increased risk of autism. There are still more questions than answers, and I appreciate that so many families are looking for answers from the scientific community.

My colleagues and supervisors at the CDC have been entirely professional since this matter became public. In fact, I received a performance-based award after this story came out. I have experienced no pressure or retaliation and certainly was not escorted from the building, as some have stated." [14]

CDC: A History of Limiting Transparency

Barbara Loe Fisher of the National Vaccine Information Center comments on the lack of transparency regarding the Department of Health and Human Services and the Centers for Disease Control and Prevention:

---

[14] Morgan Verkamp, LLC. Retrieved 2014 from:
http://www.morganverkamp.com/august-27-2014-press-release-statement-of-william-w-thompson-ph-d-regarding-the-2004-article-examining-the-possibility-of-a-relationship-between-mmr-vaccine-and-autism/

"We couldn't agree more. CDC officials should not be in the business of deliberately withholding information from the public about vaccine risks that may be greater for some children than other children. [15] Unfortunately, CDC officials have a long history of limiting transparency [16] [17] and being less than honest with the American people about what it does and does not know about vaccine risks. [18] Last July, a RAND Corporation study commissioned and funded by DHHS was published proclaiming that vaccines "are very safe." [19] What was not made clear to the public was that the study was designed and peer reviewed by high-level CDC officials, including the CDC's Director of Immunization Safety.[20]

This is a big problem for parents being ordered to give their children every government recommended vaccine – no exceptions and no questions asked. [21] [22]

[15] HRSA. Vaccine Injury Compensation Program Statistics. Accessed Aug. 29, 2014.

[16] Institute of Medicine Committee on the Review of the National Immunization Program's Research Procedures and Data Sharing Program. Vaccine Safety Research, Data Access and Public Trust. Independent Review of Vaccine Safety Datalink Activities (Pg. 96.) Washington, D.C. THE NATIONAL ACADEMIES PRESS 2005.

[17] NVIC. An Inside Job: The DHHS-Funded RAND Corp. Vaccine Safety Reviews. NVIC NEWSLETTER Aug. 12, 2014.

[18] Institute of Medicine Committee to Review Adverse Effects of Vaccines. Adverse Effects of Vaccines: Evidence and Causality. Evaluating Biological Mechanisms of Adverse Events: Increased Susceptibility. Chapter 3: p. 82. Washington, DC: THE NATIONAL ACADEMIES PRESS 2012.

[19] DHHS. AHRQ Evidence Report/Technology Assessment: Safety of Vaccines Used for Routine Immunization in the United States. July 2014.

[20] Ibid. Technical Expert Panel and Peer Reviewers (pp. 5-6).

[21] Fisher BL. Reforming Vaccine Policy & Law: A Guide. NVIC 2014.

[22] Fisher BL. Leave Parents Free to Choose Vaccines: Opposing View. USA TODAY Apr. 13, 2014.

It is a conflict of interest for DHHS to be in charge of vaccine safety and also license vaccines,[23] and take money from drug companies to fast track vaccines,[24] and partner with drug companies to develop and share profits from vaccine sales,[25] and make national vaccine policies[26] that get turned into state vaccine laws[27] while also deciding which children will and will not get a vaccine injury compensation award.[28] [29]

That is too much power for one federal agency. That is putting the fox in charge of guarding the chicken coop."

---

[23] NVIC. National Vaccine Information Center Calls on FDA to Raise Vaccine Safety and Testing Labeling Standards. NVIC NEWSLETTER May 9, 2010.

[24] NVIC. Merck's Gardasil Vaccine Not Proven Safety for Little Girls. NVIC Press Release Jun 27, 2006.

[25] Federal Register. Government-Owned Inventions: Availability for Licensing (vaccine licensing). Accessed Aug. 28, 2014.

[26] Centers for Disease Control (CDC). Recommended Immunization Schedules for Persons Aged 0 Through 18 Years - United States, 2014. DHHS Jan 1, 2014.

[27] Fisher BL. NVIC Calls for Vaccine Policy and Law Reform to Protect Human and Civil Rights. NVIC NEWSLETTER May 18, 2014.

[28] Fisher BL. The Vaccine Injury Compensation Program: A Failed Experiment in Tort Reform? Presentation to Advisory Commission on Childhood Vaccines Nov. 18, 2008.

[29] Holland MS, Krakow RJ. Brief of Amici Curiae National Vaccine Information Center, Its Co-Founders and 24 other organizations in support of petitioners. In: BRUESEWITZ V. WYETH filed with Supreme Court of the United States June 1, 2010.

"It is very telling that Congress and the U.S. Supreme Court have declared that vaccines are "unavoidably unsafe" and completely shielded drug companies from vaccine injury lawsuits.[30] [31] In America, if you or your child gets hurt by a vaccine, you can't hold anyone who developed, regulated, recommended, marketed, mandated, administered or profited from the vaccine accountable in a civil court of law in front of a jury of your peers."

Parents Concerns about Vaccine Safety Legitimate

The recent statement by a CDC senior scientist admitting that vaccine risk data is being withheld from the public is just one more piece of evidence that parents' questions and concerns about vaccine safety are legitimate.

The health of our children is at stake.

Barbara Loe Fisher's concerns are well-articulated. Her mention of financial conflicts provide the reader valid reason to ask questions before assuming that governmental agencies always have children's' best interest at heart.

Some interesting statistics about vaccine manufacturers' top fifteen profit makers are as follows:

Menactra/Meningococcal polysaccharide (serogroups A, C, Y, and W-135) diphtheria toxoid conjugate vaccine
2012 sales: $735 million
2011 sales: $557 million
Developer/Sponsor: Sanofi and Sanofi Pasteur MSD [32]

Varivax/Varicella virus vaccine live

---

[30] Supreme Court of the United States. BRUESEWITZ V. WYETH No. 09-152. Justice Sotomayor with whom Justice Ginsberg joins, dissenting Feb. 22, 2011.

[31] Business Wire. National Vaccine Information Center Cites 'Betrayal' of Consumers by U.S. Supreme Court Giving Total Liability Shield to Big Pharma. NVIC Feb. 23, 2011.

[32] Genetic Engineering and Biology News. 2014 Retrieved from: http://www.genengnews.com/insight-and-intelligenceand153/top-15-vaccines-of-2012/77899844/

2012 sales: $846 million
2011 sales: $831 million
Developer/Sponsor: Merck & Co. and Sanofi Pasteur MSD [33]

Hepatitis Franchise/Hepatitis A vaccine, inactivated (Havrix); Hepatitis A inactivated and hepatitis B (recombinant) vaccine (Twinrix); Hepatitis B vaccine (recombinant)(Engerix-B)
2012 sales: $986 million
2011 sales: $1.050 billion
Developer/Sponsor: GlaxoSmithKline [34]

Influenza Fluzone vaccine, Fluzone High dose, Fluzone Intradermal/Vaxigrip/Mutagrip
2012 sales: $1.152 billion
2011 sales: $1.077 million
Developer/Sponsor: Sanofi and Sanofi Pasteur MSD [35]

Infanrix & Pediarix/Diphtheria and tetanus toxoids and acellular pertussis adsorbed, hepatitis B (recombinant) and inactivated poliovirus vaccine combined
2012 sales: $1.183 billion
2011 sales: $1.053 billion
Developer/Sponsor: GlaxoSmithKline [36]

PENTAct-HIB/Hemophilus influenzae type b polysaccharide conjugated to tetanus protein, diphtheria, tetanus, pertussis, and inactivated poliovirus vaccines (types 1, 2, and 3)
2012 sales: $1.522 billion
2011 sales: $1.496 billion
Developer/Sponsor: Sanofi and Sanofi Pasteur MSD [37]

Gardasil/Human papillomavirus quadrivalent (types 6, 11, 16, and 18) vaccine, recombinant
2012 sales: $1.900 billion

---

[33] Ibid

[34] Ibid

[35] Ibid
[36] Ibid
[37] Ibid

2011 sales: $1.445 billion
Developer/Sponsor: Merck & Co. and Sanofi Pasteur MSD [38]

Prevnar13/Pneumococcal 13-valent conjugate vaccine (diphtheria CRM197 protein)
2012 sales: $3.718 billion
2011 sales: $3.657 billion
Developer/Sponsor: Pfizer [39]

Prevnar7/Pneumococcal 7-valent conjugate vaccine [Diphtheria CRM197 protein]
2012 sales: $399 million
2011 sales: $488 million
Developer/Sponsor: Pfizer [40]

Adacel/Tetanus toxoid, reduced diphtheria toxoid and acellular pertussis vaccine, adsorbed
2012 sales: $469 million
2011 sales: $409 million
Developer/Sponsor: Sanofi and Sanofi Pasteur MSD [41]

Rotorix/Rotavirus vaccine, live, oral
2012 sales: $549 million
2011 sales: $458 million
Developer/Sponsor: GlaxoSmithKline [42]

Pneumovax23/Pneumococcal vaccine, polyvalent
2012 sales: $580 million
2011 sales: $427 million
Developer/Sponsor: Merck & Co. and Sanofi Pasteur MSD [43]

Synflorix/Pneumococcal polysaccharide conjugate vaccine (Nontypeable Haemophilus influenzae [NTHi] protein D, diphtheria or tetanus toxoid conjugates) adsorbed
2012 sales: $587 million

---

[38] Ibid
[39] Ibid
[40] Ibid
[41] Ibid
[42] Ibid
[43] Ibid

2011 sales: $534 million
Developer/Sponsor: GlaxoSmithKline [44]

RotaTeq/Rotavirus vaccine, live oral, pentavalent
2012 sales: $648 million
2011 sales: $695 million
Developer/Sponsor: Merck & Co. and Sanofi Pasteur MSD [45]

Zostavax/Zoster vaccine live
2012 sales: $651 million
2011 sales: $332 million
Developer/Sponsor: Merck & Co. and Sanofi Pasteur MSD [46]

Take note of percent year-to-year sales growth: 96.1%. This reflects Gary Goldman's research regarding the increase in post varicella vaccine shingles increase. [47]

The CDC is both a research facility as well as a public relations organization. Do these two roles represent a conflict of interest? When individuals holding administrative positions at the CDC retire and then become executives, or consultants, at pharmaceutical companies, should we pause and contemplate their vested interests?

These are the kinds of questions that we as parents need to be asking. Careful discernment is essential when we are being told that governmental agencies are looking out for our children.

---

[44] Ibid
[45] Ibid
[46] Ibid
[47] Universal varicella vaccination: Efficacy trends and effect on herpes zoster [International Journal of Toxicology, 2005 July-Aug;24(4):205-213]; The Case Against Universal Varicella Vaccination [International Journal of Toxicology, 2006 Sep-Oct;25(5):313-317].

3 IMMUNITY

I made it through anatomy and physiology in college and avoided math successfully for four years and earned a bachelor's degree with honors. I was even elected by the faculty to the honor of "most outstanding student." Prior to homeopathy school, my medical education was "in the trenches." It was self-taught and kid-taught. My children's various illnesses, catastrophes and traumas desensitized me to fevers, vomit, blood and all manner of discharges. I also love to read, and my idea of fun has always been to snuggle up with reference books, medical texts, non-fiction, even dictionaries, for entertainment.

My infertility was the first real mother of invention. I underwent two unsuccessful invitro fertilizations and survived three ectopic pregnancies. In between three foreign adoptions, I amazingly managed to give birth to a biological son.

I was 37 at the time and honestly thought I was approaching perimenopause. I had one wimpy fallopian tube left and had been told it was completely blocked. So I had accepted the fact that I would never experience pregnancy.

It wasn't until I was vomiting every morning for a week that I thought maybe I should take a pregnancy test. Why not? I'd taken no less than a few thousand in my lifetime. One more wouldn't hurt. I was speechless when it registered positive. When I heard a heartbeat a few weeks later, I was absolutely breathless.

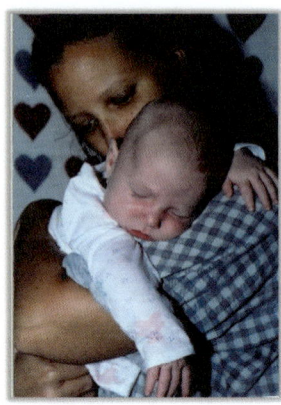

My adopted children from Taiwan (Max), China (Lily), Russia (Inga), plus homegrown Gus provided me with plenty of medical experience. Migraines, kidney reflux, ADHD, amblyopia, OCD, asthma, panic disorder and more were worrisome and time consuming. I ran through a gamut of pediatricians, specialists, prescriptions, tests and disappointments. Nothing worked for anyone!

Then a wise pediatrician on Whidbey Island in Washington made an innocent suggestion. "Why don't you try homeopathy," she said. "There are some good studies out there about its effectiveness with asthma."

I live more or less by my intuition. I just 'know' when something feels right. Homeopathy intrigued me. There was a discernable pull I was feeling. Next I made a bee line to the library where I promptly checked out some books.

I found a reputable homeopath right under my nose in Washington and made an appointment for Max. Within six months his asthma was gone. I watched as migraines also subsided and behaviors improved. I never expected kidney reflux to be impacted. But then again, never say "never."

Lily experienced recurrent kidney infections due to reflux. Reflux is when urine backs up from the bladder to the kidney by way of the ureter (the drainage tube from the kidney to the bladder). Normally, a valve between the bladder and the ureter prevents urine back washing from the bladder back into the kidney. In some children, the valve can be weak, allowing this to happen.

Fever, pain and inflammation can follow. This was the case for Lily and there was no other remedy than antibiotics. Again and again Lily developed a high fever with pain and I would know it was another kidney infection.

A few days after her first homeopathic visit she began to cry when she urinated and I knew something was up. Her fever shot up and I called her homeopath. Over the phone she asked me very specific questions about what Lily was experiencing. She then prescribed a remedy and I gave Lily a dose. Within twenty minutes her fever came down and the pain subsided. Within the next few hours, she was completely fine.

Over the next six months she would start to exhibit some symptoms as if she was getting another infection. I would give her a dose of the same remedy and it never developed into a full blown infection. No need for antibiotics. After that time, the infections never returned. And never have since. Clearly there was something about the immune system that I was discovering in a way I had never imagined.

Our Immunity

Our human immune system is quite amazing. Think of the intelligence it reflects. Day in and day out it offers protection from viruses, bacteria, parasites, and errant rogue cancer cells. It creates a balance within our biological economy of knowing when to mount a response with fever, inflammation, or discharges, and when to simply do its work silently. This elegant system actually has two distinct roles. The two arms of the immune system are called Th1 and Th2.

Th1 is responsible for cell mediated immunity, a response that does not involve antibodies, but instead activates phagocytes, antigen-specific cytotoxic T-lymphocytes, and the release of various cytokines in response to an antigen, or disease substance. This enables you to mount a fever, raising the body temperature in order to eliminate invaders.

Th2 governs the antibody-mediated response, also called the humoral ("humor" is an archaic medical term for body fluid) response. It identifies pathogens in the lymph fluid or blood and creates an inflammatory response to scavenge the offenders and eliminate them.

These two arms need to operate in a balanced way. It's essential to have an inflammatory response (Th2) in the event of radical invasion. And it's also necessary to have the constant balancing vigilance of the cell mediated (Th1) immunity.

Working in tandem, these functions mature and develop as a child matures. Nature intended for us to possess both functions. Think of them as the twenty-four hour vigilance patrol, accompanied by the emergency response team.

The emergency response function (Th2) produces antibodies. This is the goal of vaccines. In fact, they contain something called an adjuvant, from the Latin word meaning "to help," that boosts the production of antibodies. In so doing this, the inflammatory response is heightened. Think of what this means in the system of a child who has a predisposition to asthma or allergies. These two conditions are already essentially increased inflammatory responses.

Or consider the fact that whatever is contained in the vaccine ingredients will also, in the presence of an adjuvant, be perceived by the body to be a trigger to an inflammatory response. So the peanut oil, antibiotics, aluminum, formaldehyde, MSG, and other chemicals that many vaccines contain [48] will also elicit an allergic response when encountered in a child's environment or diet.

Holistically and Metaphysically

Another, more metaphysical way to view the immune system is as an overarching ability to accurately determine what is "self" and what is "not self." [49] There is no distinction inside the womb as the infant is attached by an umbilical cord to the mother. They exist as one.

---

[48] Centers for Disease Control and Prevention. (2014, Sept 10). Centers for Disease Control and Prevention. Retrieved from http://www.cdc.gov/vaccines/vac-gen/additives.htm

[49] Birch, K. & Whatcott, C., (2012) The Solution Homeoprophylaxis the Vaccine Alternative. Minneapolis: Balboa Press.

Mother's immunity is passed onto the child after he is born. Breastfeeding continues to provide protection through antibodies in mother's milk.

The separation of the birth process is the beginning of differentiation into a separate being. Some have conjectured that the first three months of life, when mother and baby are still so closely connected through nursing, is actually akin to the "fourth trimester." He cries and magically the breast appears. He is tired or fussy and there is Mother with warmth and comfort. There is little differentiation between "self" and "mother," the author of comfort.

Slowly, differentiation occurs. When uncomfortable, Baby discovers how to self soothe, perhaps with a thumb or hearing soft music. He discovers siblings can be entertaining, or is fascinated by the family pet walking by. There is a world outside himself and Mother.

At the same time, his immune system is becoming accustomed to new bacteria and viruses. Whatever he ingests first goes past the mucous membranes of his mouth, throat and intestines. Here is where innate, or natural immunity starts. These tissues contain enzymes that are antibacterial. If these tissues are penetrated by pathogens, special cells called macrophages and neutrophils respond to engulf and kill the pathogens. [50] This, along with what he breathes in, passing through the mucosa of the respiratory tract, is Baby's first encounter with what he accepts as safe for himself and what is rejected as not safe.

Fast forward to around age two when Baby learns to say, "No!" He is coming into his personal power and discerning that he is a separate person who can control what he wants and doesn't want. He practices and practices until his parents almost lose their patience in the presence of junior exercising his ability to choose. He punctuates his newfound free agency with frequent exclamations of, "Mine!"

It doesn't end here. The developing immune system continues to express itself through the maturation of social and intellectual skills in the pursuit of complete sovereignty. Any parent of a teenager can attest to the sixteen year old who is wildly independent at one moment and completely dependent the next.

---

[50] Todar's Online Textbook of Bacteriology. (Sept 2014). Retrieved from: http://textbookofbacteriology.net/innate_2.html

Every leap of independence is another illustration of the immune system determining appropriate boundaries – physically, intellectually and socially.

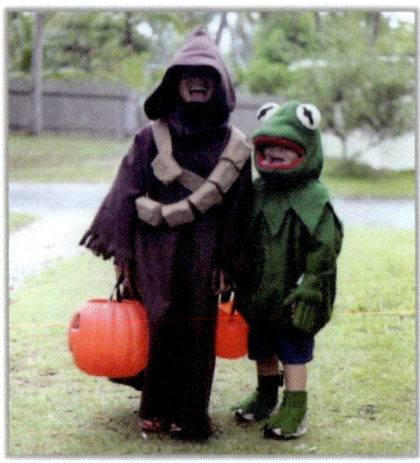

So the healthy, functioning immune system keeps us well physically, but also helps us in the ongoing process of clear boundaries, development of the personality, and differentiation between what is defined as "me" and what is "not me." Quite an amazing process, really.

It's important to understand this complex and unfolding process because true health is not just a matter of producing antibodies to specific diseases. Health occurs in human beings as a multi-faceted process. The World Health Organization (WHO) defines health as "a state of complete physical, mental and social well-being, not merely an absence of disease or infirmity, with an ability to lead to a socially and economically productive life."

We can see the relationship between physical maturation and other forms of development quite clearly in acute illness. When a child is sick and mounts a fever and has a discharge, we often see a developmental leap following resolution of the illness. They take a few wobbly steps, or learn to ride their bike, or master new words. When an older child resolves an illness, we can see leaps in independence or responsibility or problem solving skills.

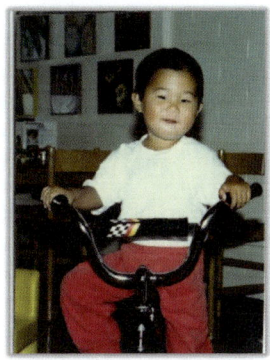

Chronic vs Acute Illness

It's important to understand the difference between chronic and acute illnesses. Chronic illness is something we rarely saw in children prior to the last few decades. Diabetes, Crohns Disease, Rheumatoid arthritis. These chronic diseases are indications of an immune system not functioning properly.

Acute disease has a beginning, a middle, and an end. We see the fussiness indicating what's called the prodromal period. Then comes a chill, followed by a fever. This is when the body is mounting an immune response. Next there is a discharge or eruption of some sort – perhaps a runny nose, a cough or the lesions of chicken pox or another virus. The fever may increase again as the body creates the final push to move towards resolution. There may be a drenching sweat and then the fever returns to normal and the entire cycle has completed. In the book, *The Solution*, we have shown a diagram of this circular immune response. [51] (also see

---

[51] Birch, K. & Whatcott, C., (2012) The Solution Homeoprophylaxis the Vaccine

diagram on page 62)

This repeated process depicts the healthy functioning of the immune system in an acute illness. Acute illnesses are nature's way of keeping the body healthy. Exercising the immune system in this way provides a vent to prevent deeper disease patterns from taking hold and developing. A fever is the body's way of cleaning out the system and resetting.

Chronic disease is the accumulation of unresolved pathology that is suppressed over time and goes deeper and deeper into the system. Circumventing the system's natural response (using something like a steroid) serves to cover the symptom and make it temporarily disappear. In reality, the unresolved pathology is only driven deeper to reemerge at another time or in another tissue or organ. We see this in cases of cancer where the initial tumor is removed, radiation and chemotherapy applied and the cancer is seemingly eradicated. But in time another malignancy crops up to be addressed – a clear indication that cancer is a systemic disease. It isn't just cut out or burned away. The system must find balance to survive.

The following diagram illustrates how long term suppression of symptoms can have a compromising effect upon the system as a whole. A misguided attempt to eliminate symptoms only drives them deeper, eliciting more serious pathology over time. Steroid creams, antibiotics, vaccinations can all seem like an immediate solution when infants manifest very common and typical childhood ailments. But as you can see in the diagram, symptoms coming from the more surface or discharging organs (such as ears or skin) can be suppressed in an attempt to relieve symptoms. This can result in pathology to deeper organs such as the lungs (asthma), digestive organs, or ultimately the nervous system.

Homeopathic medicines, or other natural methods, allow the system to stay in motion, continually seeking homeostasis and moving in the direction of improved vitality. The perceived reduction of symptoms is a false solution and ultimately stagnates the system at the expense of true health.

Alternative. Minneapolis: Balboa Press.

THERE IS A CHOICE: HOMEOPROPHYLAXIS

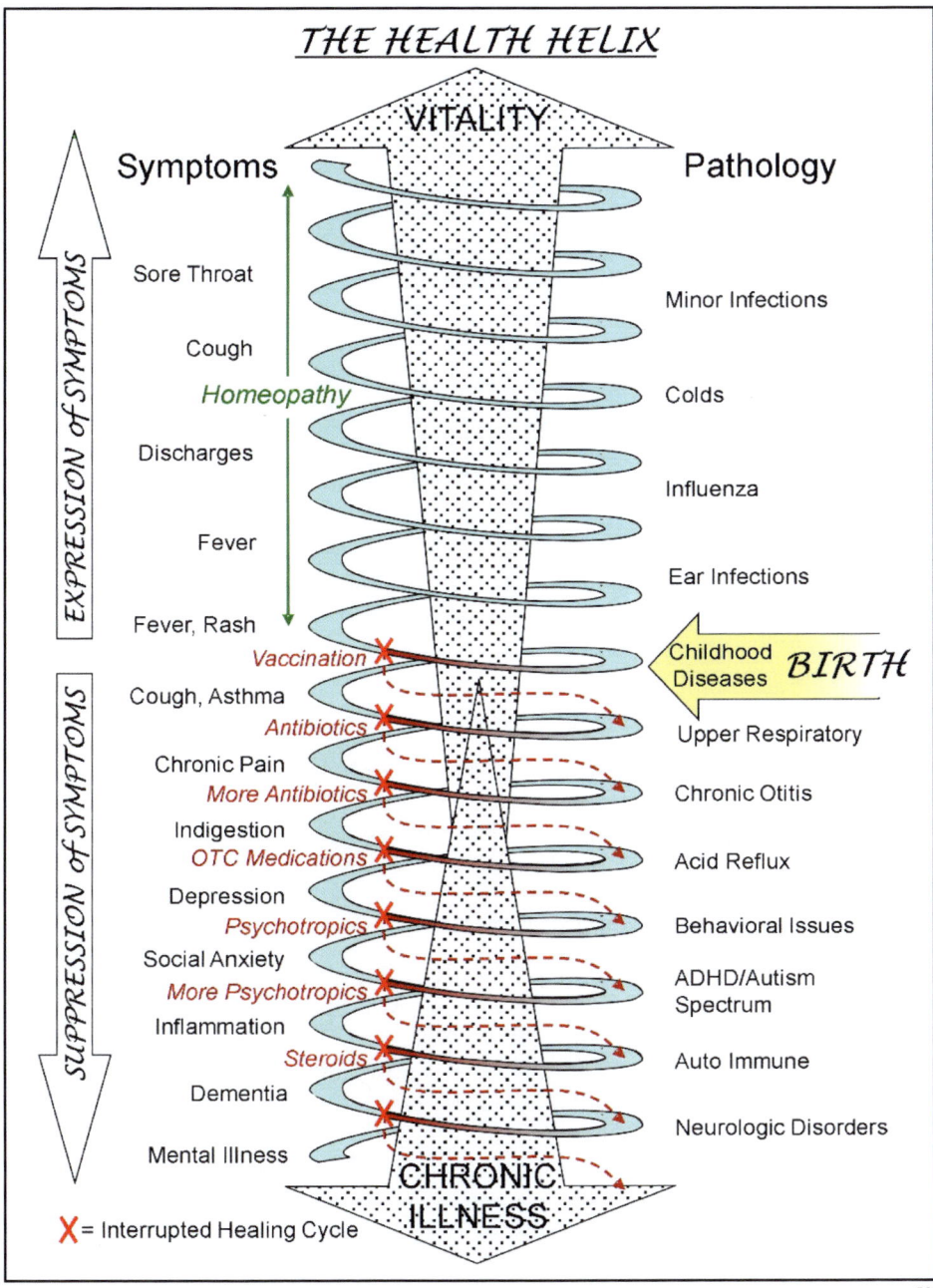

Symptoms are nothing more than expressions of the whole organism in an

[52] Neal R. Whatcott

attempt to correct itself and to find its balance to survive and flourish. When we listen to the expression and address it in a holistic way, there's an entirely different outcome. We are designed, as human beings, to expand and grow and to survive. We are programmed to self-heal, given the right environment and ingredients – love, nurturing, nutrition, stimulation and challenges. Our immune systems are attuned to this process. Our development as an individual - physically, emotionally and socially is a part of the process. Acute disease, getting sick and getting well, is an integral part of the necessary process as well. So where do bacteria, viruses and diseases fit into the picture?

Bacteria in the Big Picture

We as a human family are finally gaining the awareness that we share this planet with other life forms. No longer do we assume we have the right to control all other forms of life. The extinction of certain species has become apparent. We have exhibited great hubris over prior generations by raping the oceans, polluting the atmosphere and ravaging the earth. We are finally beginning to wake up. Part of this awakening is the understanding that bacteria and viruses are viable forms of life. And life ultimately "finds a way." It will not easily be annihilated.

Living in harmony with other forms of life is far more effective than trying to wipe out those we deem unacceptable. Do you know how many bacteria cells live in and on our body? Three to five pounds according to Lita Proctor, the program coordinator of the National Institutes of Health's Human Microbiome Project, which studies the communities of bacteria living on and in us. The bacteria cells in our body outnumber human cells 10 to 1. [53]

Do we really imagine that hand sanitizer is the answer? The solution lies in a harmonious relationship with these microbes. They assist us and we provide a host for them. Normal bacteria found in the intestine, female genital tract and oral cavity help prevent overgrowth of potential pathogens and aid digestion. [54] Bacteria are the only living things which can fix nitrogen. They are therefore essential to all other life on Earth. Developing

[53] Popular Science (Sept 2014). Retrieved from: http://www.popsci.com/science/article/2011-09/fyi-how-much-bacteria-do-people-carry-around.

[54] Life Materials Technologies Limited. (Sept 2014). Retrieved from: http://www.life-materials.com/microbes-and-human-life.html.

another antibiotic or another vaccine is not the answer.

When penicillin was introduced in the 1940's it was a wonder drug. Modern medicine had found the answer to disease. Kill the bacteria. What could be more effective and efficient than wiping out the culprits to ear infections, sore throats, wound infections and the like? Yet, today the Center for Disease Control and Prevention along with the American Academy of Pediatrics state that antibiotic resistant infections, or super bugs, are one of the world's most pressing public health threats. [55]

The medical community is now suspiciously eyeing those who choose not to vaccinate as the vector of disease.

Are the Unvaccinated Causing a Problem?

Some believe that the choice to not vaccinate a child is impacting the community in a negative way. Claims abound that disease outbreaks are due to the percentage of unvaccinated children. These children are viewed with suspicion and distrust as if they are intentionally inflicting others with diseases that they somehow manage to avoid but pass along to others.

According to the New England Journal of Medicine, a mumps outbreak during 2009 and 2010 occurred primarily among fully vaccinated children. [56]

Furthermore, getting a flu shot can have little effectiveness and actually compromise one's immunity. In the Journal of Clinical Infectious Diseases a study was described where "over a period of 9 months TIV (trivalent inactivated vaccine) recipients had increased risk of virologically-confirmed non-influenza infections Being protected against influenza, TIV recipients may lack temporary non-specific immunity that protect against other respiratory viruses." [57]

---

[55] Centers for Disease Control and Prevention. (2014). Retrieved from: http://www.cdc.gov/getsmart/

[56] New England Journal of Medicine. (Nov 2012). Retrieved from: http://www.nejm.org/doi/full/10.1056/NEJMoa1202865.

[57] Journal of Clinical Infectious Diseases 2012;54(12):1778–83. Increased risk of non-influenza respiratory virus infections associated with receipt of inactivated influenza vaccine.

This is precisely the consequence of misbalancing the Th1 and Th2 functions of the immune system. By focusing on enhancing the development of antibodies, general immunity can be compromised. And general immunity is what keeps us well in the long run.

Infant Mortality Rates

If we take a closer look at infant mortality rates, known as IMR and the relationship to rates of vaccination, a number of questions arise. The United States has the highest number of recommended vaccines in the first year of life. In 2014 that number is comprised of 30-31 doses of fourteen different diseases before age one. [58]

Thirty three other nations have a lower IMR than the United States. [59] Singapore, Sweden, Japan, Iceland, and France have some of the lowest IMR's. If vaccines are the solution for lowering disease incidence and improving infant mortality rates, why are these disturbing figures coming from mainstream medical journals?

We are all in agreement that keeping our children healthy is the top priority. And secondly, being a responsible member of the community is also a consideration. To date, vaccine marketing has instructed us that this is the only choice we have. My own research has taught me that vaccines are not the primary tool to accomplish these ends.

---

[58] Centers for Disease Control and Prevention. (2014). Retrieved from: http://www.cdc.gov/vaccines/schedules/downloads/child/0-18yrs-schedule.pdf

[59] Miller NZ, Goldman GS. Infant mortality rates regressed against number of vaccine doses routinely given: Is there a biochemical or synergistic toxicity? Human and Experimental Toxicology. 30(0) 1420-1428.

4 VACCINE STUDIES

My intention in writing this book is not to dissuade anyone from vaccinating their child. I'm simply sharing my own journey and some of the discoveries I made that led me to where I am now.

I became a fervent researcher when I realized that the responsibility for my children rested upon me. A parent is "on call" twenty four hours a day. Everyone else punches a clock. Who knows, understands and loves your child as you do? The devotion of a parent is insurmountable and immeasurable. We make the best possible decisions with the information we have at the time.

The discussion about vaccinating has become heated and emotional. One is reluctant to even broach the topic in the company of other parents. It's scarier than bringing up religion or politics! I noticed early on that those in favor of vaccination could become very emotionally heightened if challenged. They held rigidly to the concept that trust in their doctor is paramount and that the Center for Disease Control has their best interest in mind.

Their fervor is tough to debate due to the commonly held belief that vaccines are the single major reason that childhood disease has declined. I found this very curious especially when I found documentation in medical journals that disputed this assumption.

> "The largest historical decrease in morbidity and mortality caused by infectious disease was experienced not with the modern antibiotic and vaccination era, but after the introduction of clean water and effective sewer systems."[60]

More questions were raised for me regarding the additives in vaccines. Can aluminum, preservatives, adjuvents and other foreign materials really be beneficial when injected into a developing immune system? So I searched some more and this is what I found.

Here is an abbreviated list of additives such as detergents, preservatives, fixatives and antibiotics found in vaccines:

- Formaldehyde
- Polysorbate 80
- Thimerosal
- 2-phenoxyethanol
- Neomycin
- Gentamycin
- Polymixin B
- Streptomycin
- Sodium deoxycholate
- FD&C Yellow #6 aluminum lake dye

Also:

- human-diploid fibroblast cell cultures (WI-38)
- MRC-5
- Meuller's Growth Medium

Polysorbate 80 and sodium deoxycholate are known to weaken the blood brain barrier. This means they cross that protective barrier that nature created to protect developing brains. [61]

The adjuvents that can be contained in vaccines are:

- Aluminum

---

[60] Journal of Pediatrics. Dec 1999. Vol 135:no 6; pages 661-664.

[61] National Institute of Health. Retrieved from: http://www.ncbi.nlm.nih.gov/pubmed/1935140

- Monosodium glutamate
- Oil emulsions
- Squalene
- Aluminum hydroxide with monophosphoryl lipid A

Also included in vaccine manufacturing are stabilizers such as sugars, amino acids and proteins. The proteins can be human serum albumin, calf serum, monkey kidneys or porcine tissue. What hidden viruses may be in these protein sources is completely unknown.

A child receives the bulk of toxins in the first year of life. They may not show signs of toxicity until the second year because it's stored in bone and tissues and then mobilized with a febrile illness, or a fever, such as when they receive the MMR vaccine and spike a temperature. This sounds like common sense to me.

I also found volumes of studies done regarding mercury, known as thimerosal and other additives on the developing brain. Of course I delved deeper to see who conducted the study, who funded the study and also asked the question, "Does this entity have anything to gain by arriving at these results?" You should do the same in your investigations. Any study that's funded by a pharmaceutical company is suspect. Pharma has a lot to gain.

Sanofi made $5.54 billion in 2012. Sanofi makes two of the top-selling vaccines and well as Pentacel, HiB, DPT, a polio and Fluzone/Vaxigrip, a seasonal flu shot. [62]

Merck's revenue in 2012 was $5.27 billion. They make the new Gardasil vaccine for the human papilloma virus. [63]

GlaxoSmithKline brought in $5.62 billion in 2012. Early in 2014, the company signed a deal with India's Biological E to create a shot that combines its polio vaccine with a Biological E vaccine that protects against diphtheria, tetanus, whooping cough, hepatitis B and Haemophilus influenzae type b. [64]

---

[62] 2014. Retrieved from: http://www.fiercevaccines.com/special-reports/sanofi

[63] 2014. Retrieved from: http://www.fiercevaccines.com/special-reports/merck

[64] 2014. Retrieved from: http://www.fiercevaccines.com/special-

Following the breadcrumbs becomes eye-opening and downright scary. I could write an entire book on what I found. In fact, others have. But for the benefit of those who are seeking some solid evidence to share with your friends who trust their doctors unquestioningly when they say vaccines are totally safe, I've summarized some reputable studies that can easily be referenced.

Studies Regarding Vaccine Safety

The inclusion of aluminum in vaccines increased significantly when thimerosal (mercury) was reduced or eliminated. Studies by the National Institute of Health have explored the toxicity of aluminum in pediatric populations. [65] There have been questions regarding aluminum leading to auto-immune disorders. [66]

Does aluminum lead to neuron degeneration.[67] Is it associated with cognitive dysfunction? [68]

Ultimately, is it possible that aluminum could be a factor leading to autism spectrum disorders? [69]

Studies, raising frightening questions about the inclusion of thimerosal in

reports/glaxosmithkline

[65] Aluminum Vaccine Adjuvants: Are they Safe? 2014. Retrieved from: http://www.ncbi.nlm.nih.gov/pubmed/21568886

[66] Mechanisms of aluminum adjuvant toxicity and autoimmunity in pediatric populations. 2014. Retrieved from: http://lup.sagepub.com/content/21/2/223.short

[67] Aluminum hydroxide injections lead to motor deficits and motor neuron degeneration. 2014. Retrieved from: http://www.ncbi.nlm.nih.gov/pmc/articles/PMC2819810/

[68] Long-term Persistence of Vaccine-Derived Aluminum Hydroxide is Associated with Chronic Cognitive Dysfunction. 2014. Retrieved from: http://www.sciencedirect.com/science/article/pii/S0162013409001895

[69] Do aluminum vaccine adjuvants contribute to the rising prevalence of autism? 2014. Retrieved from: http://www.ncbi.nlm.nih.gov/pubmed/22099159

vaccines are coming out of National Institute of Health. [70] Mercury levels have never been completely eliminated from some vaccines. Studies have been conducted measuring the levels of methylmercury in the brains of infant monkeys given the recommended schedule. We see that toxic mercury levels can cause encephalopathy, or inflammation of the brain, and this can result in regressive symptoms of autism, [71] neurodevelopmental disorders, [72] and/or behavioral impairments. [73]

Is it wise to be exposing pregnant women to thimerosal in flu vaccines that are untested in this population? Studies show us that maternal exposure can result in a host of abnormalities for the infant? [74] Why would obstetricians recommend flu vaccines to pregnant women when there are "unavoidable risks" as stated by the CDC and no safety standards set for this population? Furthermore, the European Centre for Disease Prevention and Control states, "No European studies published in 2000 and after could be retrieved that contained data on influenza vaccine effectiveness or safety in pregnant women." [75]

---

[70] Comparison of blood and brain mercury levels in infant monkeys exposed to methylmercury or vaccines containing thimerosal. 2014. Retrieved from: http://www.ncbi.nlm.nih.gov/pubmed/16079072

[71] A Case Series of Children with Apparent Mercury Toxic Encephalopathies Manifesting with Clinical Symptoms of Regressive Autistic Disorders. 2014. Retrieved from:
http://www.ncbi.nlm.nih.gov/pubmed/17454560

[72] Neurodevelopmental disorders following thimerosal-containing childhood immunizations: a follow-up analysis. 2014. Retrieved from:
http://www.ncbi.nlm.nih.gov/pubmed/15764492

[73] Persistent behavioral impairments and alterations of brain dopamine system after early postnatal administration of thimerosal in rats. 2014. Retrieved from:
http://www.ncbi.nlm.nih.gov/pubmed/21549155

[74] Maternal thimerosal exposure results in aberrant cerebellar oxidative stress, thyroid hormone metabolism, and motor behavior in rat pups; sex- and strain-dependent effects. 2014. Retrieved from:
http://www.ncbi.nlm.nih.gov/pubmed/22015705

[75] ECDC TECHNICAL REPORT: ECDC scientific advice on seasonal influenza vaccination of children and pregnant women2014. Retrieved from:
http://www.ecdc.europa.eu/en/publications/Publications/Seasonal%20influenza%20vaccination%20of%20children%20and%20pregnant%20women.pdf

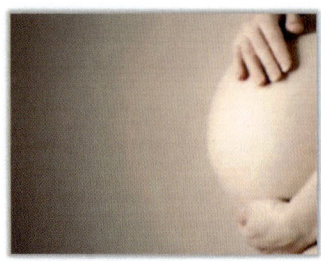

Studies have been done on rats and results show that effects to the prefrontal cortex of the brain are caused by thimerosal. [76] With infants and children there have been interesting findings in the brains, bowels and spinal fluid of those given the MMR (measles, mumps, rubella) vaccine,[77] and the association with autism disorders. [78]

The Greater Boston Physicians for Social Responsibility wrote a report on the environmental influences upon development and the specific vulnerabilities of children. Included is information on the dangerous cumulative effects of mercury, PCB's, dioxin and more. [79]

Adjuvants are meant to boost the effectiveness of vaccines and prolong the immunological response. While aluminum is one type of adjuvant, oils are also used in the form of Freund's emulsified oil, mineral oil, emulsified peanut oil (adjuvant 65), and squalene (shark oil). [80]

---

[76] Administration of thimerosal to infant rats increases overflow of glutamate and aspartate in the prefrontal cortex: protective role of dehydroepiandrosterone sulfate. 2014. Retrieved from: http://www.ncbi.nlm.nih.gov/pmc/articles/PMC3264864/?tool=pubmed

[77] Abnormal measles-mumps-rubella antibodies and CNS autoimmunity in children with autism. 2014. Retrieved from: http://www.ncbi.nlm.nih.gov/pubmed/12145534

[78] Serological association of measles virus and human herpesvirus-6 with brain autoantibodies in autism. 2014. Retrieved from: http://www.ncbi.nlm.nih.gov/pubmed/9756729

[79] In Harm's Way: Toxic Threats to Child Development. 2014. Retrieved from: http://action.psr.org/site/DocServer/frontmatter.pdf?docID=5121

[80] Scheibner, V PhD. Adverse Effects of Adjuvents in Vaccines. Nexus Dec 2000

Viera Schneiber, PhD from the Slovak Republic makes the following statement:

> "According to Gupta et al. (1993), the toxicity of adjuvants can be ascribed in part to the unintended stimulation of various mechanisms of the immune response. That's why the safety and adjuvancy must be balanced to get the maximum immune stimulation with minimum side effects."
>
> She continues by saying, "My conclusion is that such balance is impossible to achieve, even if we fully understood the immune system and the full spectrum of deleterious effects of foreign antigens and other toxic substances such as vaccine and drug adjuvants and medications on the immune systems of humans, and particularly on the immature immune systems of babies and small children. Injecting any foreign substance straight into the bloodstream will only cause anaphylactic (sensitisation) reactions."[81]

Vol 8, No1 & Feb 2001 Vol 8, Number 2.

[81] Ibid.

Numerous studies associate vaccines with encephalopathy and subsequent autistic disorders. [82] [83] [84] [85] [86] [87] [88] This is what my daughter, Lily, experienced after receiving multiple vaccines at one time. Fortunately, she recovered completely and did not regress to autistic spectrum symptoms.

---

[82] A Case Series of Children with Apparent Mercury Toxic Encephalopathies Manifesting with Clinical Symptoms of Regressive Autistic Disorders. 2014. Retrieved from:
http://www.ncbi.nlm.nih.gov/pubmed/17454560

[83] Acute disseminated encephalomyelitis. 2014. Retrieved from:
http://www.neurology.org/content/68/16_suppl_2/S23.abstract

[84] Acute necrotizing encephalopathy secondary to diphtheria, tetanus toxoid and whole-cell pertussis vaccination: diffusion-weighted imaging and proton MR spectroscopy findings. 2014. Retrieved from:
http://www.springerlink.com/content/44xt417387hx4877/

[85] Encephalo-Myelitis following Vaccination. 2014. Retrieved from:
http://www.ncbi.nlm.nih.gov/pmc/articles/PMC2047920/

[86] Acute encephalopathy and chronic neurological damage after pertussis vaccine. 2014. Retrieved from:
http://www.ncbi.nlm.nih.gov/pubmed/7906066

[87] The smallpox vaccine and postvaccinal encephalitis. 2014. Retrieved from:
http://www.ncbi.nlm.nih.gov/pubmed/12170398

[88] Encephalopathies following prophylactic pertussis vaccine. 2014. Retrieved from: http://pediatrics.aappublications.org/content/1/4/437.abstract

Severe encephalitis can result in death. The Journal of American Medicine reported on deaths subsequent to the smallpox vaccine between 1959 and 1968. [89] Acute encephalopathy continued to cause brain damage in infants from the pertussis vaccine [90] as well until it was changed from a live vaccine to an acellular vaccine in 1996. [91]

Sudden Infant Death syndrome (SIDS) also known as "crib death" is a tragic occurrence that has sometimes been erroneously attributed to parental abuse, such as shaking babies violently. This is termed "shaken baby syndrome." There is evidence of vaccine induced SIDS as portrayed in some studies by the National Institute of Health and others. [92] [93] In fact, there is an interesting relationship with the increasing numbers of vaccines given to the rising infant mortality statistics in some nations. [94]

---

[89] Subacute sclerosing panencepholitis – the continuous threat. Deaths Attributable to Smallpox Vaccination, 1959 to 1966 and 1968. 2014. Retrieved from:http://jama.jamanetwork.com/article.aspx?volume=212&issue=3&page=441

[90] Acute encepholapathy and chronic neurological damage after pertussis vaccine. 2014. Retrieved from: http://www.ncbi.nlm.nih.gov/pubmed/7906066

[91] World Health Organization. 2014. Retrieved from: http://www.who.int/biologicals/vaccines/pertussis/en/

[92] Simultaneous sudden infant death syndrome. 2014 Retrieved from: http://www.ncbi.nlm.nih.gov/pubmed/17654772

[93] Unexplained cases of sudden infant death shortly after hexavalent vaccination. 2014 Retrieved from: http://www.sciencedirect.com/science/article/pii/S0264410X05004688

[94] Infant mortality rates regressed against number of vaccine doses routinely given: is there a biochemical or synergistic toxicity? 2014 Retrieved from: http://www.ncbi.nlm.nih.gov/pmc/articles/PMC3170075/

Despite claims that non-vaccinating families are the culprits in outbreaks of measles, mumps or pertussis, there are studies showing us that the opposite is actually true. Those vaccinated are contracting the diseases. [95] [96] [97]

Could it be that artificially-induced immunity is not as effective as once thought? [98] [99] [100] Or perhaps bacteria and viruses are adapting in order to survive? [101]

We also cannot ignore the growing possibility, or perhaps the inevitability, that vaccines can very likely become contaminated in the manufacturing process. [102] [103] [104]

---

[95] Measles outbreak in a fully immunized secondary-school population. 2014 Retrieved from: http://www.ncbi.nlm.nih.gov/pubmed/3821823

[96] Mumps outbreak among vaccinated university students associated with a large party, the Netherlands, 2010. 2014 Retrieved from: http://www.sciencedirect.com/science/article/pii/S0264410X12006299

[97] Risk of vaccine failure after Haemophilus influenzae type b (Hib) combination vaccines with acellular pertussis. 2014 Retrieved from: http://www.thelancet.com/journals/lancet/article/PIIS0140-6736(03)13171-6/fulltext

[98] Why Do Pertussis Vaccines Fail? 2014 Retrieved from: http://pediatrics.aappublications.org/content/129/5/968.extract

[99] Waning Protection after Fifth Dose of Acellular Pertussis Vaccine in Children. 2014 Retrieved from:http://www.nejm.org/doi/full/10.1056/NEJMoa1200850

[100] Unexpectedly limited durability of immunity following acellular pertussis vaccination in preadolescents in a North American outbreak. 2014. Retrieved from: http://cid.oxfordjournals.org/content/54/12/1730.abstract

[101] Recent Resurgence of Mumps in the United States. 2014 Retrieved from: http://www.nejm.org/doi/full/10.1056/NEJMoa0706589#t=article

[102] The Dangerous Impurities of Vaccines. 2014 Retrieved from: http://www.scribd.com/patrons99/d/49973741-Dangerous-Impurities

[103] Adventitious Agents and Vaccines. 2014 Retrieved from: http://www.ncbi.nlm.nih.gov/pmc/articles/PMC2631857/pdf/11485673.pdf

This calls to mind whether questionable science is applied to vaccine development. [105] And how are we to view legal policies that are rolled out to protect manufacturers above consumers? [106] The Advisory Council on Immunization Policy (ACIP) recommends all pregnant women be vaccinated against the flu, yet this is not supported in current medical literature. [107] In a critical assessment of the ACIP's recommendations, David Ayoub, MD and Edward Yazbak, MD state in their conclusion,

> "The ACIP's recommendation of influenza vaccination during pregnancy is not supported by citations in its own policy paper or in current medical literature. Considering the potential risks of maternal and fetal mercury exposure, the administration of thimerosal during pregnancy is both unjustified and unwise. Pregnancy should continue to be a time when doctors are highly protective of their patients with regard to any fetal exposure. Without adequate safety testing, a risk-benefit analysis of influenza vaccination during pregnancy is not possible, and therefore the ACIP's present recommendation should be withdrawn." [108]

In fact, the seasonal influenza vaccine was only recently added to the recommended schedule. Prior to 2010 it was only recommended for elderly populations.[109] Those elderly were housed in communal settings such as nursing homes where the risk of contamination was high. Under the age of fifty, mortality is negligible. [110]

---

[104] Quantitation of DNA and Protein Impurities in Biopharmaceuticals -Liver Cancer? 2014 Retrieved from:
http://pubs.acs.org/doi/abs/10.1021/ac00009a003

[105] Adverse Effects of Vaccines: Evidence and Causality. 2014 Retrieved from:
http://www.iom.edu/Reports/2011/Adverse-Effects-of-Vaccines-Evidence-and-Causality.aspx

[106] Human papillomavirus (HPV) vaccine policy and evidence-based medicine: Are they at odds? 2014 Retrieved from:
http://informahealthcare.com/doi/abs/10.3109/07853890.2011.645353

[107] Influenza Vaccination During Pregnancy: A Critical Assessment of the Recommendations of the Advisory Committee on Immunization Practices (ACIP) 2014 Retrieved from:
http://www.jpands.org/vol11no2/ayoub.pdf

[108] Ibid.

The recommendation for babies (6 months old) to receive flu vaccines has caused increased adverse events resulting in suspension of vaccinating young children in some nations. [111]

In conclusion, we are well aware that drug trials and experimentation have taken place without the knowledge of recipients in places like Tuskegee, [112] Africa, [113] India [114] and Guatemala. [115] What other trials may have been conducted, or are currently being conducted, without public knowledge or consent from recipients?

---

[109] 2014 Retrieved from:
http://www.immunize.org/askexperts/experts_inf.asp

[110] Excess mortality from seasonal influenza is negligible below the age of 50 in Israel: implications for vaccine policy. 2014 Retrieved from:
http://www.springerlink.com/content/2p44p50005827585/

[111] Australia suspends seasonal flu vaccination of young children. 2014 Retrieved from:
http://www.bmj.com/rapid-response/2011/11/02/adverse-events-following-influenza-vaccination-australia-should-we-be-surp

[112] Centers for Disease Control and Prevention. 2014 Retrieved from:
http://www.cdc.gov/tuskegee/timeline.htm

[113] Age of autism. 2014 Retrieved from:
http://www.ageofautism.com/2014/09/minority-report-a-covert-cdc-program-inoculated-black-babies-with-deadly-experimental-measles-vaccines.html

[114] Human papillomavirus vaccine trials in India. 2014 Retrieved from:
http://www.thelancet.com/journals/lancet/article/PIIS0140-6736(11)60270-5/fulltext

[115] National Public Radio. 2014 Retrieved from:
http://www.npr.org/blogs/health/2010/10/01/130266301/u-s-apologizes-for-medical-research-that-infected-guatemalans-with-syphilis

5 HOMEOPROPHYLAXIS

So what would be effective, contain no additives, chemicals or preservatives, be easy to administer, inexpensive and easily distributed?

Homeoprophylaxis is the answer.

Homeoprophylaxis is the use of diluted and potentized disease products, called "nosodes," as well as other potentized natural substances to elicit an immune response. This response may not produce antibodies, but it will educate the immune system in a way that has been clinically shown to reduce the incidence of both infectious as well as chronic disease.

Where did it originate? How does it work? Is it really safe? Will it work for my children? These are the questions that any responsible parent would ask.

First let's talk about how to say it. It's pronounced Home-e-o-pro-phyl-axis. Emphasis is on the syllable "pro." It may be a mouthful, but it's actually a very simple concept. The word will be rolling off your tongue easily by the end of this chapter. We also call it "HP" for short.

Homeoprophylaxis has been around for a very long time. It's been utilized in multiple countries – India, Brazil, Cuba, the United States, Europe,

Australia and many others. When I first heard of it, I was intrigued and started my research. Eventually in the discovery process, something just clicked for me. It made perfect sense. Here's how it began.

In the Beginning

Samuel Hahnemann, MD (1755-1843), the father of homeopathy, was treating a family with four children in 1801 when three of them contracted scarlet fever. The fourth child, who was under his care for something else had been taking homeopathic (diluted and succussed to contain no remaining molecules) Belladonna. This fourth child never contracted scarlet fever. Hahnemann deduced that the Belladonna was acting preventatively.

His next opportunity to see if this was an accurate deduction was when three children in a family of eight were stricken with scarlet fever. He immediately gave the five well children Belladonna. None of the five fell ill, despite exposure to their siblings. His hypothesis was correct! This was a remarkable result when the attack rate of scarlet fever was 90%. [116]

The Practice Gained Popularity

Other conventional physicians, or allopaths, then began to use Belladonna effectively and word spread quickly that this was an effective prophylaxis. Cristoph Hufeland, described as the greatest German clinician of the late 18th century, supported the use of Belladonna as a prophylactic enthusiastically. His endorsement was so influential that the Prussian Government then made its use during scarlet fever epidemics obligatory in 1838, [117] two years after Hufeland's death.

Contributing to the endorsement of Belladonna as an effective homeoprophylactic was an article published in *The Lancet* in 1829, by Cristoph Hufeland (1762–1836), reporting the following:

> "The proper use of belladonna has, in most cases, prevented infection, even in those instances where, by the continual intercourse with patients labouring under scarlet fever, the predisposition towards it was greatly increased.

[116] Dudgeon, Lectures on the Theory and Practice of Homeopathy, Republished by Archibel, Encyclopedia Homeopathica, July 2000.

[117] Dunham, Caroll. Lectures on Materia Medica, Republished by Archibel, Encyclopedia Homeopathica, July 2000.

Numerous observations have shown that, by the general use of belladonna, epidemics of scarlet fever have actually been arrested.

In those few instances where the use of belladonna was insufficient to prevent infection, the disease has been invariably slight.

There are exceptions to the above three points, but their number is extremely small." [118]

What is it?

Let's first start with an explanation of homeopathy. The word "homeo" means "similar." "Pathy" means "pain." Homeopathy is derived from "like" curing "like." In other words, a substance which can cause certain symptoms, will also cure similar symptoms. This is the same concept used by Hippocrates (460-350 B.C), the father of modern medicine. He stated: *"By similar things a disease is produced and through the application of the like, it is cured."*

For example, if a child fell ill with seizures, the plant called henbane could be given. Henbane causes seizures and Hippocrates knew that it could possibly cure the child as well. Unfortunately, the child could also die from too strong a dose.

It was Dr. Samuel Hahnemann- a scientist, physician and linguist, who determined that diluting and succussing the original substance could capture the healing effects while rendering it harmless and removing any risk.

In the dilution process, no molecules of the original substance remain after the twelfth round of dilution and succussion. Over and over again, one drop of the original substance is added to ninety-nine drops of a solution. This serial dilution process is central to potentizing the medicinal effects of remedies. With this method, even highly poisonous substances, such as snake venoms, poisonous plants, or toxic metals could be utilized for their curative properties.

Moreover, with each dilution the entire bottle is succussed. Succussion is accomplished by firmly impacting the bottle against a hard surface. In doing

---

[118] Hufeland M. On the prophylactic powers of belladonna against scarlet fever. Lancet 1829;1:135.

so, the dynamic energetic nature of the original substance is potentized.

Another example would be the use of highly poisonous bee venom as a remedy. If stung by a bee and the area is becoming hot, red and swollen, you can take apis mellifica, homeopathically prepared bee venom, and your symptoms will quickly subside. Your own body is responding to the introduction of the apis in a curative manner.

When remedies have been homeopathically prepared in this very specific manner of dilution and succussion, remedies are non-toxic and at the same time highly effective and curative.

Some people find it implausible that homeopathic medicines, diluted past any molecular content, can have any effect. Cutting edge studies show us how an "ultra molecular" dilution is capable of storing energetic information from the substance it has previously been in contact with. [119]

What about Homeoprophylaxis?

Homeoprophylaxis works in a slightly different way. Instead of waiting for symptoms to arise, HP can be given prior to contact with an infectious disease. It has been shown to protect from targeted diseases just as Samuel Hahnemann found Belladonna could protect during the scarlet fever epidemic. Many such remedies used are produced in FDA approved homeopathic pharmacies.

Nosodes are made from substances of the targeted disease. Biological discharges, such as sputum, or exudates are used as the original substance. The solution is then serially diluted and potentized in the same way as explained above.

This process is a type of "attenuation." Attenuation means to "weaken" and a similar process is used in manufacturing conventional vaccines. With vaccines, though, there is still some of the original disease product present after attenuation. This is the "antigen" found in any vaccine. This is the first of a few key differences between HP and vaccination.

The most obvious difference is the purity of the homeopathic nosodes compared to conventional vaccines. The homeopathic

[119] Delinic AN, Physical properties of water and how they relate to homoeopathic preparations. In Proceedings of the 9th Hellenic Medical Homoeopathic Conference. Athens. May 1993.

nosodes contain no additives whatsoever. **No antibiotics, no preservatives, no detergents, no foreign DNA, or unknown viruses are present in HP nosodes.**

With our increased awareness of the hazards of environmental toxicity, this fact alone is remarkable. Do we want to knowingly inject known carcinogens into developing immune systems? Can we trust that "trace" amounts of aluminum or mercury or monosodium glutamate are as harmless as we are told?

I don't know how sensitive your children are, but my own were so highly attuned to the slightest change in their diet or environment that I could tell by their behavior exactly what they had eaten in the last twenty four hours. Given something like monosodium glutamate, I could see the results in a matter of minutes!

Injections

It occurred to me early on that taking a child to the doctor for a vaccine was laden with high anxiety. Mostly my own! Restraining a screaming baby or child while the nurse zoomed in with empty reassurances that "this won't hurt a bit," somehow didn't feel like great parenting.

Perhaps I was having flashbacks to my own childhood. Tearfully recovering from the sting of the needle after a shot was administered, I reluctantly accepted the proffered lollypop as a consolation prize. After a cursory glance at the shiny round treat, I heaved it across the room at the nurse as hard as I could!

As a homeopath, I later understood that the natural transmission of infectious disease is through coughing, sneezing, or contact with body fluids. In this manner, the first exposure we have occurs through contact with mucous membranes. This is where immune cells reside and begin their initial work in responding to disease. [120]

Bypassing the respiratory tract by injecting a substance directly into the blood stream is like an ambush attack to the immune system. There is no opportunity to mount a preliminary response in a biologically natural and appropriate way.

Homeopathic nosodes are administered on small sugar pellets. They

[120] Immunology. Mar 1971; 20(3): 277–288.

dissolve on the tongue and enter the system by way of the natural route past mucous membrane. Here the natural process of disease recognition can begin in the way that Mother Nature intended.

Why So Many Shots?

I stood in line for a sugar cube. It was 1959 and my mother loaded me into the sedan to drive to the elementary school. We waited in a long line for a tiny paper cup containing a harmless looking little sugar cube. The wait held no anxiety. I had been assured there were no shots involved. Upon the cube was a drop of something to keep me safe from catching a disease called polio.

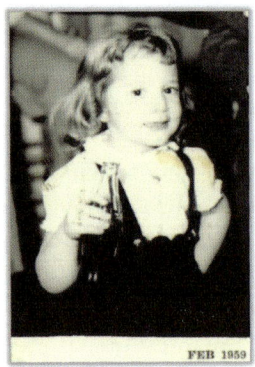

Yours Truly

I was happy to pop it into my mouth. The delicious sweetness slowly melted on my tongue and I happily went back home to play with little concern that I had just partaken in a bit of history – human vaccine trials.
This particular polio vaccine, the Sabin attenuated poliovirus, was offered in human trials conducted until 1962 when it was then licensed.

Other than this dose of polio vaccine, I received one dose of DPT, (diphtheria, pertussis, tetanus) and no other vaccines. I did receive multiple doses of penicillin, once for an abscessed tooth and a few other times for illnesses. It was the wonder drug that eliminated infection at the time and it was liberally administered. It was either one of these shots, or the DPT, that precipitated my dramatic candy-flinging performance at Dr. Tilly's office.

I recall having both mumps and chicken pox before the age of ten. These events were occasions to stay home from school, drink lots of ginger ale, have my temperature taken at regular intervals, and partake of bonus television time.

Most of my friends had these illnesses too. It was accepted as a rite of passage during early grade school years. It never seemed terribly serious and we were back to school on the playground within a week or so, comparing chicken pox scars or what indulgences we enjoyed during our individual convalescence. The real prize we were unaware of at the time, was the lifelong immunity we had just acquired in exchange for a week of illness.

Today's Vaccine Schedule

In 2014 children are immunized with approximately thirty doses of disease by the time of their first birthday. [121] Many of the shots combined multiple diseases in single injections such as the DTaP (diphtheria, acellular pertussis, tetanus), or the MMR (measles, mumps, rubella), or the quadruple dose of MMRV (with added varicella) or perhaps the Pentacel with five different diseases included (diphtheria, pertussis, tetanus, polio and Haemophilis B influenza).

Why have so many shots been added to the schedule? Young moms today are under the impression that all of these recommended vaccines have always been the norm. That is not so.

The official annual schedule endorsed by the Advisory Committee on Immunization Practices (ACIP), the American Academy of Pediatrics (AAP), and the American Academy of Family Physicians (AAFP).did not appear until 1995. [122] Prior to that time, the smallpox vaccine was used in the 1940's. The DTP was also recommended at that time, but not officially required for school attendance. In the late 1950's, the polio vaccine was added, first as the Salk live form and later the Sabin attenuated form.

It wasn't until the 1970's that the MMR was officially recommended making the total number of recommended vaccines to total seven diseases, causing it to look like this:
- Tetanus
- Diphtheria

---

[121] Centers for Disease Control and Prevention. Retrieved from: www.cdc.gov

[122] College of Physicians of Philadelphia. Retrieved from: http://www.historyofvaccines.org/content/articles/development-immunization-schedule

- Pertussis (whooping cough)
- Polio
- Measles
- Mumps
- Rubella [123]

Since the late 1980's Rotovirus, Pneumonia, Haemophilis B, Meningitis, annual Influenza, Hepatitis A, Hepatitis B, Varicella and Human Papilloma virus have been included, making the recommended list to now look like this:

- Hepatitis B
- Rotavirus
- Diphtheria, Tetanus, and Pertussis (combined DTaP vaccine)
- Hib (*Haemophilus influenzae* type b)
- Pneumococcal
- Polio (inactivated vaccine)
- Influenza
- Measles, Mumps, and Rubella (combined MMR vaccine)
- Varicella (chickenpox)
- Hepatitis A
- Meningococcal
- Human Papilloma Virus (HPV)

My own generation was the first to be regularly vaccinated and I received shots for just four diseases I mentioned: polio, diphtheria, pertussis and tetanus.

"Booster" shots were not necessarily required at that time. The next generation of children born in the 1970's/1980's received vaccines for about seven diseases. These were all communicable diseases. They were considered epidemic in nature and could cause death or lasting effects.

The following generations born in the 1990's and beyond were welcomed with the prospect of being vaccinated against disease prior to epidemic contamination. In other words, a pre-emptive strike was launched on non-epidemic diseases such as Hepatitis A and B, Rotovirus, and HPV. In third

---

[123] Ibid.

world countries these diseases can be dangerous when there is little access to sanitary conditions or clean water, but in the United States they are not considered to be epidemics, nor life-threatening.

Hepatitis

Hepatitis A is a communicable disease that is transmitted through the oral-fecal route. It can be transmitted by restaurant workers who don't wash hands after using the restroom, or other food sources. Outbreaks can also occur from sewage-contaminated water. Symptoms usually include nausea, malaise, fever, abdominal pain, darkened urine and jaundice. It can last up to two months. 10% of people can have symptoms for up to six months. The fatality rate is between two and three percent of those who contract it.

Hepatitis B is a viral infection that attacks the liver and can become chronic. It is passed by sharing blood products or body fluids. It can also be passed from mother to child at birth. In the early 1990's it became the recommendation to give this vaccine on the day of birth in the U.S. without testing the mother first to determine if she was a carrier.

The incidence of Hepatitis B in the United States is less than 1%. [124] Less than 5% of healthy adults who contract it will develop a chronic infection.[125] Chronic infection can be a concern. Chronic disease happens when the immune system is compromised or the symptoms are suppressed in such a way as to drive them deeper into the individual. 15–25% of adults who develop this chronic infection during childhood can die from hepatitis B-related liver cancer or cirrhosis. [126]

---

[124] Mediacentre. (2014) Retrieved from: http://www.who.int/mediacentre/factsheets/fs204/en/

[125] Ibid.

[126] Ibid.

Rotovirus

There are multiple types of rotovirus and it's possible to be infected multiple times. [127] The most common form is rotovirus A. Just about every child in the world has been infected by rotovirus at least once by the age of five. [128] It is a common childhood illness. The route of transmission is by oral-fecal contamination.

The symptoms include possible fever, stomach pain and watery diarrhea. In developing countries where there is little access to clean water, dehydration can be a cause of death. In the United States there are only 1.6 to 2.3 deaths per 100,000 cases annually. [129]

Human Papillomavirus

In 2009 I attended a conference sponsored by the National Vaccine Information Center. While there I heard Diane Harper, MD, MPH speak about her experience as one of the leading experts on the human papillomavirus. Merck Pharmaceutical had consulted with her during the development of the Gardasil vaccine. At the NVIC 4th International Conference she shared some valuable information.

---

[127] Mayo Clinic. Retrieved from: http://www.mayoclinic.org/diseases-conditions/rotavirus/basics/causes/con-20026103

[128] Bernstein DI (March 2009). "Rotavirus overview". The Pediatric Infectious Disease Journal 28 (3 Suppl): S50–3.

[129] Esposito DH, Holman RC, Haberling DL, Tate JE, Podewils LJ, Glass RI, Parashar U. Pediatr Infect Dis J. 2011 Nov; 30(11):942-7.

It wasn't until 1976 that a link was discovered between the human papillomavirus and cervical cancer. There are thirteen high risk strains that cause 70% of cervical cancers. Dr. Harper made it clear that the Gardasil vaccine did not prevent cancer, per se. It simply targeted four strains of HPV "6, 11, 16 and 18."

She expressed the importance of pap screening as it detects very early pre-cancers. She states that pap screening does not kill or handicap. [130] She also shares publicly that if the duration of protection is fifteen years, then vaccinating 11-year-old girls will only protect them until they are 26. If duration of efficacy is less than fifteen years, then no cancers are prevented, only postponed. [131]

Most sexually active women contract HPV. It can only be spread by transmission of blood or lymph through a tear in the tissue. 60% of sexually active women are infected with it. It's very slow growing, taking 5-30 years to progress to cancer. 70% of cases resolve spontaneously in one year and 90% of all cases resolve spontaneously within two years. [132] This tells us that a healthy immune system is capable of resolving HPV long before it develops into cancer. Detected early, the cure rate is 93%. [133]

---

[130] Huffington Post Interview. Retrieved from: http://www.huffingtonpost.com/marcia-g-yerman/an-interview-with-dr-dian_b_405472.html

[131] Ibid.

[132] Diane Harper, MD. 4th International Public Conference on Vaccination. NVIC. 2 October 2009

[133] American Cancer Society. (2014). Retrieved from: http://www.cancer.org/cancer/cervicalcancer/detailedguide/cervical-cancer-survival

Furthermore, there is at least one verified case of auto-immune initiated motor neuron disease declared triggered by Gardasil presented by neurologists at the 2009 American Neurological Association meeting in Baltimore, Maryland. [134]

At least one state, Utah, has excluded it from their public health clinics. When asked why this was excluded, Dr. David Blodgett of the Salt Lake Public Health Department responded that Gardasil was fast tracked through the FDA and that Merck was overselling the benefits. [135]

One must question if these vaccines, Hepatitis A and B, Rotovirus and HPV vaccine, are really necessary interventions. Do the risks outweigh the benefits? What is the risk of death from these diseases? Are the diseases they address considered epidemic? And why so many diseases at once? Are we really powerless against all childhood diseases as well as those that stem from a developing disease process?

How does homeoprophylaxis address these questions?

One Disease at a Time

The developing immune system manages one disease at a time effectively. If a child is sick, it is best to allow him to get well before introducing any other diseases to his system. Most medical professionals would say it is inadvisable to be giving a vaccine at that time, until he is well. The Center for Disease Control and Prevention states that you should not vaccinate your child if he is "moderately or severely sick, with or without a fever." [136]

---

[134] Huffington Post Interview. (2014) Retrieved from: http://www.huffingtonpost.com/marcia-g-yerman/an-interview-with-dr-dian_b_405472.html

[135] Blodgett, D Salt Lake Tribune. Retrieved October 3, 2014 from: http://healthimpactnews.com/2013/utah-health-official-bans-gardasil-vaccine/

[136] Centers for Disease Control and Prevention. (2014) Retrieved from: http://www.cdc.gov/vaccines/recs/vac-admin/contraindications-vacc.htm

I would add that giving multiple doses of different antigens in the form of combination vaccines may be fraught with complications. Allowing the body to mount a complete response to one disease at a time is the most beneficial. Let's define a complete response.

When we come into contact with a contagious disease there is a prodromal period. This is prior to any symptoms becoming obvious. Next there is a slight rise in body temperature. This can be perceived as chills and achiness. The immune system has become engaged in the process. Several types of cells then work together to recognize the disease (or antigen) and respond. B lymphocytes and T lymphocytes seek out the foreign substance, lock onto it and try to rid the body of the foreigner.

This is when we can see inflammation and systems or tissues begin to discharge. Next there is a discharge. Perhaps there's a rash, or some other physical manifestation. We can see this as a cough, a runny nose, or a throbbing ear infection. The last stage is when the fever can mount, resulting in a drenching sweat before the entire process is resolved and health is restored.

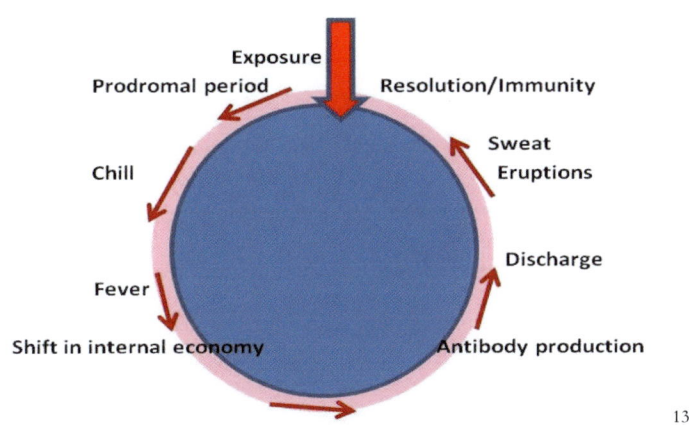

This is where homeoprophylaxis shines. Only one disease is introduced to the body at a time. This allows the immune system to mount a response and resolve the disease effectively. In the case of childhood diseases, only those communicable diseases that pose a risk are typically given.

---

[137] Birch, K, Whatcott, C. (2012) The Solution: Homeoprophylaxis The Vaccine Alternative. Minneapolis. Balboa Press

To summarize, homeoprophylaxis, or HP, is a disease prevention method that uses diluted and potentized disease particles. It respects the immune system by only introducing one disease at a time through a natural route of administration passing through mucous membrane.

The HP nosodes contain no adjuvents, no preservatives, no antibiotics, no detergents, and are not grown on mediums such as animal tissues that contain foreign DNA or unknown viruses.

HP has been utilized since the 1800's and was even made obligatory by the Prussian government in 1838 during scarlet fever outbreaks. It is commonly used for epidemic diseases that pose the risk of death or disability, but can also be used for diseases with a low mortality rate, or when traveling to an area where a specific disease is endemic.

The benefit of homeoprophylaxis is that it "educates the immune system" in such a way as to either protect from the disease, or if it's contracted, an asymptomatic or mildly symptomatic case will occur.

6 HISTORICAL EVIDENCE

Since the 1800's many cases of scarlet fever, cholera, smallpox, polio, pertussis, measles, mumps, chicken pox, diphtheria, Japanese encephalitis, dengue fever, typhoid, influenza, meningitis and more have been successfully cured or prevented by the use of homeopathy and homeoprophylaxis.

There were seven separate pandemics of cholera ranging from 1817-1961 killing tens of millions of people. Clemens von Boenninghausen both prevented and cured large numbers of individuals with cholera during the 1949 epidemic using homeopathy and homeoprophylaxis.

The death rate with conventional medicine, which consisted of boiling drinking water and sufficient rehydration, was as high as 90% at that time. Boenninghausen's patients had a mortality rate of only 5%-16%. [138]

---

[138] Von Boenninghausen, C. Baron.1984. Bönninghausens Kleine medizinische Schriften [Lesser Medical Writings] (ed. Klaus H. Gypser), Heidelberg, 1984.

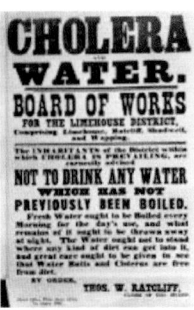

Diphtheria

Diphtheria was a highly feared childhood disease caused by a bacteria called c. diphtheriae and characterized by a leathery, sheath-like membrane that grows on the tonsils, throat and in the nose. The word, dipthera, is Greek for leather.

The HP nosode, diphtheriinum was used for Diphtheria in France by Chavanon in 1932. Many children produced antibodies, as detected by the Schick test, a simple procedure for measurement of specific diphtheria antibodies which is no longer used.[139] This suggested that their immune systems had possibly mounted this response as a result of coming in contact with the disease after receiving HP. This is what is meant by "educating the immune system." [140]

Poliomyelitis

Reaching a peak in the 1940's and 1950's, polio was a feared disease that afflicted 500,000 people worldwide. Symptoms included fever, headache, vomiting, fatigue, muscle soreness or stiffness and subsequent paralysis. [141]

Treatments ranged from oxygen, hydrotherapy, electrotherapy, and herbal poultices to braces and iron lungs. Quarantines were put in place for homes where a family member was afflicted. Violating the quarantine or removing

---

[139] Sullivan, JL, Herrod, HG, Levine, L. The Schick Test. A Useful Tool for Screening for Antibody Deficiency. Am J Dis Child. 1981 Jul; 135(7):618-20. Retrieved 2014 from: http://www.ncbi.nlm.nih.gov/pubmed/7018216

[140] Chavanon, P. 1952. La Dipterie, 4th Ed, St Denis, Niort: Imprimerie.

[141] Mayo Clinic (2014) Retrieved from: http://www.mayoclinic.org/diseases-conditions/polio/basics/symptoms/con-20030957

the posted placard was punishable by up to a costly $100 fine in the early 1900's. [142]

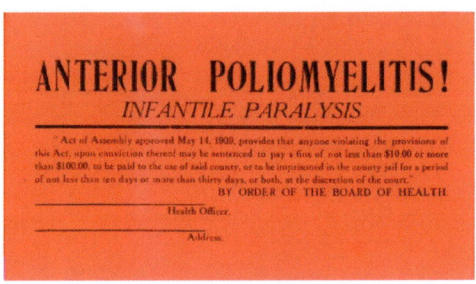

Many people have vivid memories of this epidemic and personal experiences. My close friend, Diane, grew up with her mother who had been stricken by polio and was confined to a wheelchair. Diane recalls always helping to clean the dust from tops of cupboards and door jambs, or places her mother could not reach from her chair.

Between 1956 and 1958, Dr. H. Heisfelder used Lathyrus sativus for prophylaxis of polio for over 6,000 children. There were no side effects and no cases of polio reported in the group. [143]

In 1957 and again in 1975 there were severe outbreaks of polio in Buenos Aries, Brazil. Dr. Francisco Eizayaga also used the homeopathic remedy Lathyrus sativus as a prophylactic for over 40,000 people. Pharmacies distributed thousands of doses to the public. There were no further cases of contagion registered. [144]

An American MD and homeopath, Arthur Grimmer reported outstanding results in the 1950's using Lathyrus for the prevention of polio. Some reports state that he protected over 30,000 individuals. [145]

---

[142] Wikipedia (2014) Retrieved from: http://en.wikipedia.org/wiki/History_of_poliomyelitis

[143] Eisfelder, HW. Poliomyelitis Immunization: A Final Report. Journal of the American Institute of Homeopathy. V. 54, Nov-Dec 1961, pp. 166-167.

[144] Francisco Eizayaga MD. Treatise on Homeopathic Medicine published by Ediciones Maracel, Buenos Aires, Brazil, 1991

[145] Currim, Ahmed N., Ed., The Collected Works of Arthur Hill Grimmer, M.D., Hahnemann International Institute for Homeopathic Documentation, Norwalk

Pertussis

Whooping cough is a highly contagious bacterial disease that results in paralysis of respiratory cells that lead to inflammation in the respiratory tract. It is most threatening to very young babies and less symptomatic in adults.

Dr. Dorothy Shepherd claimed 100% protection by using the HP nosode called pertussin. She states, "I used it for years in the nurseries, in my private practice, in the medical clinic, and in hundreds of cases in various epidemics we went through, and truly it is a great remedy." [146]

The 1918 Spanish Influenza

The Spanish influenza epidemic of 1918 and 1919 was also called "La Grippe." It first appeared in the late spring of 1918 and was fairly mild. In the following fall it returned with a vengeance and people were showing symptoms in the morning and falling dead by evening. The death toll was higher than that of World War I. An estimated 30-40 million people succumbed.

The war was winding down during this time and peace was on the horizon. What initially seemed like a benign cold surfaced amongst pockets of people. Because patients experienced symptoms not traditionally associated with influenza, physicians found the disease especially difficult to diagnose in the early stages of the pandemic. Many physicians and scientists even claimed that influenza patients were suffering from cholera or bubonic plague, not influenza.

---

and Greifenberg, 1996.

[146] Shepherd, D., (1967). Homeopathy in epidemic diseases (First ed.). Essex, England: The C. W. Daniel Company Limited. p.18.

Early symptoms included a temperature between 102 and 104 degrees Fahrenheit. Patients also experienced a sore throat, exhaustion, headache, aching limbs, bloodshot eyes, a cough and occasionally a violent nosebleed. Some suffered from digestive symptoms such as vomiting or diarrhea. Many patients recovered only to suffer a relapse. Their temperatures, which had fallen, rose again and they now experienced serious respiratory problems. In some cases, these patients also experienced massive pulmonary hemorrhages. After death, pathologists found these victims to have swollen lungs and oversized spleens. [147]

This "cold" was most deadly for those between the ages of twenty and forty. This was an unusual occurrence for influenza, which usually impacts infants and the elderly the hardest.

Noted in the Journal of The American Medical Association in late 1918:

> "The 1918 has gone: a year momentous as the termination of the most cruel war in the annals of the human race; a year which marked, the end at least for a time, of man's destruction of man; unfortunately a year in which developed a most fatal infectious disease causing the death of hundreds of thousands of human beings. Medical science for four and one-half years devoted itself to putting men on the firing line and keeping them there. Now it must turn with its whole might to combating the greatest enemy of all-- infectious disease." Dec 1918 [148]

Those 20-40 year olds with vibrant immune systems were falling dead from the Spanish Flu most rapidly. The ravages of WWI placing additional stress on immune systems, and the widespread travel of troops across continents were surely contributing factors. One explanation to the failure of "modern medicine" as a cure could possibly be explained by the discovery of one of the first pharmaceutical drugs.

In 1897, about twenty years earlier, Felix Hoffmann of the Bayer pharmaceutical company developed the process of synthesizing the acetyl salicylic acid later named "aspirin." Aspirin was considered a wonder drug for reducing fever, pain and inflammation.

[147] U.S. Department of Health and Human Services. 2014. Retrieved from: http://www.flu.gov/pandemic/history/1918/the_pandemic/fightinginfluenza/index.html

[148] Retrieved from: https://virus.stanford.edu/uda/ 2014.

Naturally, aspirin was freely distributed in hopes of reducing the fever. Suppressing the body's natural defense of a fever seemed to backfire in cases resulting in a sudden turn for the worse. Aspirin also thins the blood and hemorrhage was one of the telltale signs that death was near as the flu raged. While aspirin reduced the uncomfortable fever, giving a false sense of improvement, it also increased the hemorrhagic tendency of the respiratory tract.

Homeopaths were not using aspirin. Instead they were gathering the symptoms of the cases before them and prescribing remedies that most closely matched. Their cure rate was unsurpassed! "Old school" medical treatment of aspirin had a mortality rate of 28%-30%. Homeopathy had a mere 1.05% of patients die. [149]

Dr. T A McCann, from Dayton, Ohio reported that 24,000 cases of flu treated allopathically had a mortality rate of 28.2% while 26,000 cases of flu treated homeopathically had a mortality rate of 1.05%. This figure was supported by Dean W.A. Pearson of the Philadelphia Medical School, also known as Hahnemann College, who collected 26,795 cases of flu treated with homeopathy. [150]

Conventional Modern Flu Shots

Influenza immunizations only recently became recommended for infants starting at the age of six months in 2004. [151] Prior to that time, flu shots were predominantly utilized by the elderly living in communal settings such as nursing homes.

According to the Centers for Disease Control and Prevention flu vaccines contain the following excipients and mediums:

- Monosodium glutamate
- Polysorbate 80

[149] Bradford, Thomas, MD (1900). The Logic of Figures. Philadelphia, PA. Boericke and Tafel.

[150] National Center for Homeopathy 2014. Retrieved from: http://www.homeopathycenter.org/treatment-epidemics-homeopathy-history

[151] College of Physicians of Philadelphia. 2014. Retrieved from: http://www.historyofvaccines.org/content/articles/influenza

- Formaldehyde
- Thimerosal
- EDTA
- Antibiotics
    - Gentamicin
    - Neomycyn
    - Polymyxin
- Foreign proteins [152]

Monosodium glutamate (MSG) has been shown to cause multiple side effects, including difficulty breathing, headache, diarrhea, mood changes, dizziness, sleep problems and more. Furthermore, evidence of subsequent brain lesions and endocrine disorders are evident. Olney et al. (New England Journal of Medicine) points out that neurotoxic effects of monosodium glutamate and its related amino acids have been well documented. [153]

Polysorbate 80 is a chemical that can cross the blood brain barrier. This is the barrier that nature put in place to protect developing brains. It should not be accessed by chemicals. The Toxicology Data Network has this to say: "Polysorbates have also been associated with serious adverse effects, including some deaths, in low birth weight infants intravenously administered a vitamin E preparation containing a mixture of polysorbates 20 and 80." [154]

Formaldehyde is a known carcinogen according to the National Cancer Institute. [155]

Much has been said about **thimerosal,** including the claim that it is absolutely safe to inject into infants. It was removed from many vaccine in

---

[152] Centers for Disease Control and Prevention. 2014. Vaccine Excipient & Media Summary. Excipients included in US vaccines. Updated 2013.

[153] Olney JW, Ho OL, Rhee V, De Gubareff T. Neurotoxic effects of glutamate. New Engl J Med. 1973; 289(25):1374-1375.

[154] Rowe, R.C., Sheskey, P.J., Quinn, M.E.; (Eds.), Handbook of Pharmaceutical Excipients 6th edition Pharmaceutical Press, London, England 2009, p. 551-3

[155] National Cancer Institute. 2014. Retrieved from: http://www.cancer.gov/cancertopics/factsheet/Risk/formaldehyde

1999 but remains in trace amounts in influenza vaccines.

EDTA stands for ethylene diamine tetraacetic acid. EDTA is a penetration enhancer. That means that it breaks down the tissue's protective barrier, making it easier for other potentially harmful ingredients in the formula to sink deeper into tissues and the bloodstream. EDTA is cytotoxic and genotoxic, meaning it is toxic to living cells and genetic material such as DNA. [156]

Antibiotics are being used in vaccine production to help prevent bacterial contamination during manufacturing. [157] Alexander Fleming, who won a Nobel Prize for his discovery of penicillin, warned that misuse of the drug could result in selection for resistant bacteria. [158]

Inappropriate use of antibiotics has been recognized and warned against very recently by the Academy of Pediatrics. Antibiotics have no effect on viral infections such as the common cold. They are also ineffective against sore throats, which are usually viral and self-resolving. [159] Most cases of coughs are viral as well, passing after a few weeks. The use of antibiotics against these is unnecessary and can put children at risk of suffering adverse reactions. [160]

Long Term Health

Risks of other illnesses are increased with the use of flu vaccines. A study

[156] Lanigan, RS, Yamarik, TA. Final report on the safety assessment of EDTA, calcium disodium EDTA, diammonium EDTA, dipotassium EDTA, disodium EDTA. Int J Toxicol. 2002;21 Suppl 2:95-142.

[157] Department of Health and Human Services. 2014. Retrieved from: http://www.fda.gov/BiologicsBloodVaccines/SafetyAvailability/VaccineSafety/ucm187810.htm

[158] Environ Health Perspect. Jun 2009; 117(6): A244–A250.

[159] Little P, Gould C, Williamson I, Warner G, Gantley M, Kinmonth AL (August 1997). "Reattendance and complications in a randomised trial of prescribing strategies for sore throat: the medicalising effect of prescribing antibiotics." BMJ 315 (7104): 350.

[160] Hueston WJ (March 1997). "Antibiotics: neither cost effective nor 'cough' effective". The Journal of Family Practice 44 (3): 261–5.

done in 2012 revealed that the use of influenza vaccine actually increased the risk of getting sick with other viruses. The results stated that "inactivated influenza vaccine recipients may lack temporary non-specific immunity that protects against other respiratory viruses." [161]

Long term health outcomes can be negatively compromised by flu shots as well as excessive doses of other vaccines. We know from reliable studies that a correlation was found between infant mortality rates (IMRs) and the number of vaccine doses routinely given. [162] Russell Blaylock MD, a respected neurosurgeon has elucidated the ill-effects of vaccination during brain development. [163] Harold E Buttram, MD and Catherine J Frompovich have also concurred in the International Medical Council on Vaccination. [164]

There are many studies that report poor efficacy of flu vaccines.

Cochrane Collaboration

The Cochrane Collaboration is a well-respected international not-for-profit organization preparing, maintaining and promoting the accessibility of systematic reviews of the effects of health care. Their latest review of flu vaccine efficacy states the following:

"Over 200 viruses cause influenza and "influenza-like illness" which produce the same symptoms (fever, headache, aches and pains, cough and runny noses). Without laboratory tests, doctors cannot tell the two illnesses apart. Both last for days and rarely lead to death or serious illness. At best, vaccines might be effective against only influenza A and B, which represent about 10% of all circulating viruses." [165]

---

[161] Cowling, B., Fang, V., Nishiura, H., et al. Journal of Clinical Infectious Diseases Clinical Infectious Diseases 2012;54(12):1778–83

[162] Miller, N., Goldman, G. Infant mortality rates regressed against number of vaccine doses routinely given: Is there a biochemical or synergistic toxicity? Hum Exp Toxicol. Sep 2011; 30(9): 1420–1428.

[163] Blaylock, r. MD. The Danger of Excessive Vaccination During Brain Development. Medical Veritas, 2008; 5(1): 1727-1741.

[164] International Medical Council on Vaccination. 2011. Retrieved from: http://www.vaccinationcouncil.org/2011/06/01/vaccines-and-brain-inflammation/

They go on to say: *"Authors of this review assessed all trials that compared vaccinated people with unvaccinated people. Vaccine use did not affect the number of people hospitalized or working days lost but caused one case of Guillian-Barré syndrome (a major neurological condition leading to paralysis) for every one million vaccinations. Fifteen of the 36 trials were funded by vaccine companies and four had no funding declaration."* [166]

Additionally, *"Results may be an optimistic estimate because company-sponsored influenza vaccines trials tend to produce results favorable to their products and some of the evidence comes from trials carried out in ideal viral circulation and matching conditions and because the harms evidence base is limited."* [167]

They conclude with, *"Children (< 16 years old) and the elderly (above 65 years old) are the two age groups that appear to have the most complications following an influenza infection."* [168]

---

[165] Demicheli V, Jefferson T, Al-Ansary LA, Ferroni E, Rivetti A, Di Pietrantonj C. 2014. Retrieved from: http://summaries.cochrane.org/CD001269/ARI_vaccines-to-prevent-influenza-in-healthy-adults.

[166] Ibid.

[167] Ibid.

[168] Jefferson T, Rivetti A, Di Pietrantonj C, Demicheli V, Ferroni E. 2012. Vaccines for preventing influenza in healthy children. Retrieved from: http://summaries.cochrane.org/CD004879/ARI_vaccines-for-preventing-influenza-in-healthy-children.

Studies with homeoprophylaxis for the prevention of influenza have shown positive results. [169] Homeoprophylaxis for influenza and other diseases has been used for over 200 years and no side effects or adverse reactions have ever been reported.

The World Health Organization states that homeopathy is the second most utilized system of health care in the world. In the United States, there are more than 500 physicians and 5000 non-physicians using homoeopathy in clinical practice. [170]

Furthermore, in 2003-2004, the WHO issued a 40-page draft on homoeopathy, entitled "Homoeopathy: Review and Analysis of Reports on Controlled Clinical Trials," claiming that the "majority" of peer-reviewed scientific papers published over the past 40 years "have demonstrated that homoeopathy is superior to placebo in placebo-controlled trials and is equivalent to conventional medicines in the treatment of illnesses, in both humans and animals." [171]

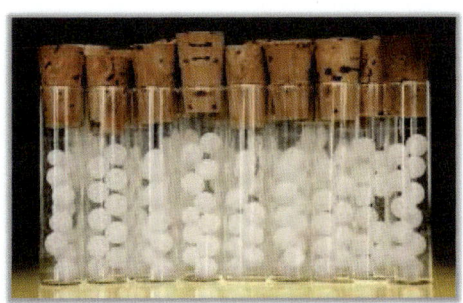

---

[169] Lyrio, C., Siqueira,C., Veiga, V., et all. The use of homeopathy to prevent symptoms of human flu and acute respiratory infections: a double-blind,randomized, placebo-controlled clinical trial with 600 children from Brazilian Public Health Service. Int J High Dilution Res 2011; 10(36):174-176

[170] Lawrence M.Tierney, Jr. et al, "Current Medical Diagnosis & Treatment", USA: The McGraw-Hill Companies, Inc. 2004 (1701-03; 4th ed.)

[171] Published by Elsevier Ltd. August 2005. The Lancet, Volume 366, Issue 9487, Pages 705 - 706

7 CURRENT EVIDENCE OF HOMEOPROPHYLAXIS

If some diseases seem like ancient history, we can also look to more modern trials of homeoprophylaxis and its accompanying success. Meningitis, Leptospirosis, many tropical diseases as well as childhood infectious diseases have been prevented since the 1970's. Some examples have been quite dramatic.

Meningitis

Bacterial meningitis is caused by any one of several bacteria. Neisseria meningitidis or "meningococcus" is common in children and young adults, and Streptococcuspneumoniae or "pneumococcus" is another common cause in children and adults. Haemophilus influenzae type b (Hib) can be a common cause of meningitis in infants and young children. Neisseria meningitidis and Streptococcuspneumoniae account for most of the bacterial meningitis cases in the U.S.

Viral meningitis is more common than the bacterial form and generally less serious. It can be triggered by a number of viruses. People with viral meningitis are much less likely to have permanent brain damage after the infection resolves. Most will recover completely. [172]

In 1974 there was an epidemic of meningitis in Brazil. Dr. Francisco Eizayaga gave 18,640 children the homeoprophylactic remedy called meningococcinum. 6,340 children were in the untreated group. In the group treated with HP only four cases of meningitis occurred. In the untreated group there were thirty two cases.

This was repeated in 1988 with individuals between the ages of 0-20 years old. The group treated with meningococcinum had 65,826 participants. In this group only one case of meningitis was reported in the following six months. Of the 25,532 untreated individuals, seven cases were reported. Twelve months later, follow-up reported three cases in the protected group and thirteen cases in the unprotected group. This works out to be eighteen times the disease attack rate in the untreated group!

Statistical analysis demonstrated homeoprophylaxis displayed 95% protection from contracting meningitis in children under six months old and 91% protection in children over 12 months old. [173]

There were no deaths, no adverse effects, and no side effects from the use of homeoprophylaxis.

The conventional meningococcal vaccine (MenHibrix, Menactra, Menomune, or Menveo) has been found to be about 58 percent effective within two to five years after adolescents receive the shot. The product inserts for meningococcal vaccine list adverse events reported during clinical trials or post licensure, including irritability, abnormal crying, fever, drowsiness, fatigue, injection site pain and swelling, sudden loss of consciousness (syncope), diarrhea, headache, joint pain, Guillian-Barré Syndrome, brain inflammation, convulsions, and facial palsy. [174]

---

[172] Centers for Disease Control and Prevention (2014) Retrieved from: http://www.cdc.gov/meningitis/index.html

[173] Mroninski C, Adriano E, Mattos G. Meningococcin, its Protective Effect against Meningococcal Disease, Homœopathic LINKS Winter, 2001 Vol 14 (4) 230-4

[174] Vaccine package insert. (2014) Retrieved from: http://www.fda.gov/downloads/BiologicsBloodVaccines/Vaccines/ApprovedProducts/UCM201349.pdf

As of August 2012, the federal Vaccine Adverse Events Reporting System (VAERS), which includes only a small fraction of the health problems that occur after vaccination in the U.S., had recorded more than 2,300 serious health problems, hospitalizations and injuries following meningococcal shots, including 39 deaths. About 40% of the deaths occurred in children under age six. [175]

Leptospirosis

Leptospirosis is a bacterial disease caused by the bacteria called leptospira. It can be carried by wild and domestic animals showing no symptoms. In humans, the symptoms can be fever, headache, chills, vomiting, jaundice, abdominal pain, and rash. There are two phases. The first manifests with fever, chills, headache, muscle aches, vomiting, or diarrhea. There can be recovery for a time but if a second phase occurs, it is more severe, with possible kidney or liver failure or meningitis. [176]

This bacterial infection is primarily seen in tropical regions where hurricanes and flooding are common. As rodents urinate in open fields, people come in contact with the standing water and can contract the disease. It is especially endemic to Cuba where the government annually vaccinates the entire population to protect against leptospirosis.

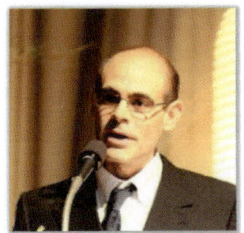

Dr. Gustavo Bracho

---

[175] National Vaccine Information Center (2014) Retrieved from: http://www.nvic.org/vaccines-and-diseases/Meningitis.aspx

[176] Centers for Disease Control and Prevention. 2014. Retrieved from: http://www.cdc.gov/leptospirosis/symptoms/index.html

Dr. Gustavo Bracho is an immunologist who works for the Carlos J. Finlay Institute, a world renowned center for vaccine research and production in Havana, Cuba. He is advisor to the President and General Director of Finlay Institute, and head of the Homeopathy and Biotherapic Projects at the Institute. He is an experienced researcher in molecular and cellular biology, and has headed the Adjuvant Group within the Immunology Department of Finlay.

Dr. Concepción Campa is a scientist, pharmacist and lead researcher at the Finlay Institute who works alongside Dr. Bracho. "Concita" as Dr. Campa is lovingly known by the people of Cuba, is well known and loved as a woman who has done outstanding work to improve the health of the population. She possesses buoyant energy, passion about her work and great motivation to serve her fellow human beings.

I had the privilege of meeting them both in Barcelona, Spain in 2013 during an international conference. They presented their findings from their study with 2.3 million individuals given homeoprophylaxis for the prevention of leptospirosis in 2007 and 2008.

The results of the study were remarkable. PubMed, a respectable source for medical research states:

> RESULTS: After the homeoprophylactic intervention a significant decrease of the disease incidence was observed in the intervention regions. No such modifications were observed in non-intervention regions. In the intervention region the incidence of Leptospirosis fell below the historic median. This observation was independent of rainfall.
>
> CONCLUSIONS: The homeoprophylactic approach was associated with a large reduction of disease incidence and control of the epidemic. The results suggest the use of HP as a feasible tool for epidemic control, further research is warranted. [177]

The following graph indicates the dramatic drop in infections in 2008 in the intervention region (IR) compared to the non-intervention region (RC) where the incidence actually rose.

---

[177] PubMed 2014. Retrieved from:
http://www.ncbi.nlm.nih.gov/pubmed/20674839 Bracho G1, Varela E, Fernández R, Ordaz B, Marzoa N, Menéndez J, García L, Gilling E, Leyva R, Rufín R, de la Torre R, Solis RL, Batista N, Borrero R, Campa C. Large-scale application of highly-diluted bacteria for Leptospirosis epidemic control. Homeopathy. 2010 Jul;99(3):156-66. doi: 10.1016/j.homp.2010.05.009.

The dotted line indicates the predicted rate of infection for the area based on historical incidence at the same time of the year. As you can see, the drop was significantly below the prior year (2007). When Dr. Bracho and Dr. Campa presented continued findings in Barcelona, they reported that cases were still below average and expected in 2012. Furthermore, the surrounding region was also experiencing a reduction of cases.

This can be understood as the morphogenetic field effect. Those in close proximity were benefiting from the effects of lowered incidence of leptospirosis, much like the concept of "herd immunity."

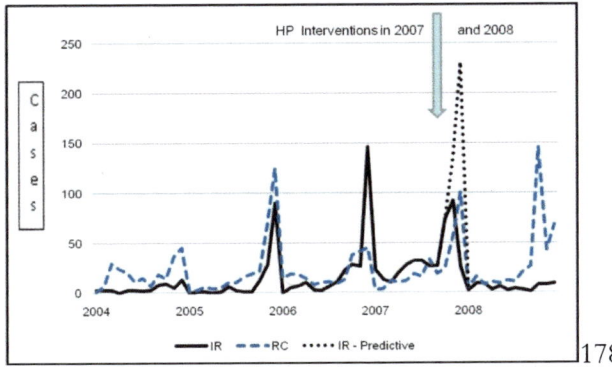[178]

Even more remarkable were the spirits of Dr. Bracho and Dr. Campa who having dedicated their lives to vaccine research, are now devoted to the exploration of homeoprophylaxis. I stole a few precious moments outside the conference with Dr. Bracho and asked him about his personal feelings regarding the leptospirosis study. In halting English and with humble demeanor he expressed his excitement about the new direction his career was taking. This discovery enlivened his passion about his work and the prospects of learning more and doing more good in the world.

Dr. Campa expressed her concern for all the children who had been vaccinated when this simple method of homeoprophylaxis is "so harmless and so effective." Her kind and gentle nature shone through her eyes as we spoke. I was deeply touched by both Dr. Campa and Dr. Bracho.

---

[178] Bracho G1, Varela E, Fernández R, Ordaz B, Marzoa N, Menéndez J, García L, Gilling E, Leyva R, Rufín R, de la Torre R, Solis RL, Batista N, Borrero R, Campa C. Large-scale application of highly-diluted bacteria for Leptospirosis epidemic control. Homeopathy. 2010 Jul;99(3):156-66.

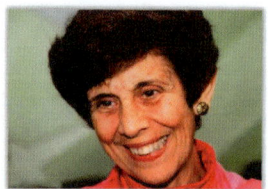

Dr. Concepción Campa

In a world where there is so much contention and disagreement on the safety and efficacy of vaccines, these two individuals had the integrity and courage to explore a different way. Not only did they explore homeoprophylaxis with open minds, they accepted a method vastly different than what they had devoted their entire careers to. This is the integrity of true scientists and humanitarians.

8 DR. ISAAC GOLDEN

Without the seminal work of Isaac Golden, this book would not be possible.

I initially met Dr. Golden by telephone during a conference call with a colleague in 2012. We maintained an email relationship for the next two years. In August of 2014, I sat across the table from Isaac in a restaurant in Toronto Canada. It was then that I saw and understood the man behind the reputation. When asked why he engaged upon his work with homeoprophylaxis, he replied, "It's my dharma."

There is no single translation for the word dharma in western languages. The classical Sanskrit meaning of the word is "to hold, maintain, or keep." In Hinduism, dharma signifies behaviors that are considered to be in accord with the order that makes life and the universe possible. For Sikhs, the word dharm means the "path of righteousness." Clearly, the concept of dharma embodies the principles of conduct, virtue, meaning and cosmic order.

I believe in cosmic order. I believe in serendipity. And I also believe that all things happen exactly when they are meant to happen, and in exactly the right way. These beliefs give me great peace.

When I first heard of Dr. Golden's work in 2009, I felt an immediate flash of recognition. I knew this work was authentic. I knew it would be instrumental in changing how we look at immunization. It was the answer to the conundrum I had seen young mothers and families facing while trying to keep their children safe.

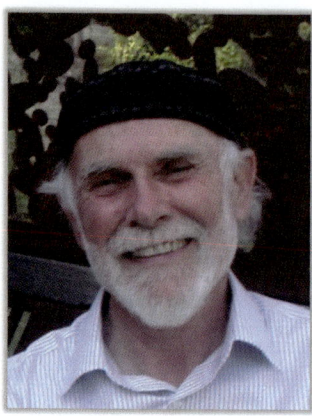

Dr. Isaac Golden

Around the same time as this flash of recognition, my colleague Kate Birch traveled to Cuba where she presented at a conference and met Dr. Golden. At that time she asked if she could bring his work to the United States.

Isaac, following his dharma, agreed and Kate returned home to create a preliminary plan to offer homeoprophylaxis to parents and at the same time collect data of their experience to further support Dr. Golden's findings.

Sometime later, at an informal meeting of homeopaths in her office, I readily agreed to join in bringing the program to parents. Kate and I subsequently wrote "The Solution: Homeoprophylaxis the Vaccine Alternative," for parents to have a book for the purpose of sharing the concept of HP with family and friends who were both curious and skeptical.

Kate and I went on to found the non-profit organization Free and Healthy Children International to promote education about HP, its distribution and the continued collection of data to validate the effectiveness of homeoprophylaxis.

Research and Studies

Dr. Golden is a pioneer. In 1985 there were no published homeoprophylaxis programs that could be used in place of the recommended childhood vaccine schedule, and no one was systematically collecting evidence to support the use of such programs. Isaac's work stands as the keystone to future applications of homeoprophylaxis for infectious childhood diseases.

While homeoprophylaxis has been utilized for over 200 years for both epidemics as well as cases of endemic contagious disease, the application as an alternative to the recommended government immunization schedule is new. It's a concept met with skepticism by some conventional medical practitioners. Having Dr. Golden's emerging evidence of effectiveness is critical to creating a grassroots movement of parents who support and appreciate the ease, safety and effectiveness of the method.

Many individuals seek out and depend upon only random controlled, double blind studies that are summarized in medical journals. Physicians are taught in school that this is the only reliable method of testing. We would like to believe that medical science is full of integrity and can be trusted to deliver accurate and verifiable information. Unfortunately, this is not always the case.

At his recent presentation in Toronto Isaac shared his opinion that "there is no such thing as a perfect study." He referenced John P. A. Ioannidis, a Professor of Health Research and Policy at Stanford School of Medicine, the University's Rehnborg Chair in Disease Prevention and director of its Prevention Research Center, and co-director of the Meta-Research Innovation Center at Stanford (METRICS). Ioannidis was chairman at the Department of Hygiene and Epidemiology, University of Ioannina School of Medicine as well as adjunct professor at Tufts University School of Medicine. He is best known for his research and published papers on scientific studies, starting with the 2005 paper "Why Most Published Research Findings Are False".[179]

---

[179] Ioannidis, J. P. A. (2005). "Why Most Published Research Findings Are False." PLoS Medicine 2 (8): e124. doi:10.1371/journal.pmed.0020124 PMC 1182327

Additionally there are multiple articles coming out of Harvard University evaluating ethics, corruption and manipulation of data. [180] Many of these are related to the pharmaceutical industry.

When people ask if there are double blind random controlled studies on homeoprophylaxis, I usually reply that those types of studies are not compatible for testing homeopathic methods. And in fact many vaccines have not been subjected to large scale RCT testing for effectiveness either (as opposed to safety) as it is not considered ethical to deny test subjects the protection of vaccines. The evidence of clinical application seems much more suitable. If something is actually working in the field, why not devise methods to extrapolate information in the most accurate way?

Some individuals criticize homeopathy for the absence of molecular substance in remedies, saying there can be no mechanism of action. Anything that deals with the non-material is viewed with suspicion. Dr. Golden shares that aspirin was used for over three decades before its mechanism of action was known. He contends that a real scientist continues to investigate when there is evidence of something working, but is not yet understood. And we see clinical evidence that homeoprophylaxis works.

Dr. Golden is careful to add that no method of disease prevention is 100% effective. There is no perfect solution – not vaccination, nor homeoprophylaxis, nor just doing nothing at all. He also states that "there is no such thing as homeopathic vaccination." Homeoprophylaxis is simply a method of immunizing against future contagious infection that would reduce the likelihood of developing symptoms if exposed to the disease. [181]

---

[180] Harvard University. Edmond Safra Center for Ethics. Retrieved from: http://ethics.harvard.edu/working-papers-series

[181] Golden, Isaac (2012). The complete Practitioner's Manual of Homeoprophylaxis. Victoria, Australia. Page xi.

Do No Harm

As parents, every decision we make for our children has consequences. Our fears far outweigh reality most of the time. I always tell my clients that if we possessed a crystal ball and could see into the future for even ten minutes to glimpse what the future held, we would sleep much more soundly at night.

As a parent and as a healer, I take very seriously my commitment to "do no harm." My deepest belief is that we are all motivated to heal. Healing takes place in a highly individualized manner. We cannot judge, predict or dictate how another will heal. Knowing this, I hold tremendous respect for others as they follow their individual path. In my efforts to do no harm, and allow others adequate space while supporting their journey, I always try to choose the path of least risk.

The choices we make for our children at times feel so risky. Surely they involve so much more than merely their physical safety. Social and emotional development are huge factors contributing to well-being. Our relationships with each child are also of utmost importance. These relationships have effects that reverberate throughout future generations.

Choosing the path of least risk often means allowing natural consequences to occur or opting for the least invasive intervention. It should always include not being coerced by fear. It is only when we are devoid of fear that our natural intuition can emerge to guide and direct us.

Long Term Health Outcomes

A very interesting finding of Dr. Golden's work is the improved long term health outcomes of children using homeoprophylaxis instead of conventional vaccination. The use of homeoprophylaxis also provided improved long term outcomes when compared with unvaccinated children who parents used a general 'make-the-child-as-healthy-as-possible' approach to infectious disease prevention.

It seems that allowing exposure to the natural disease in energetic form carries this benefit without any of the risks.

In the table below, (Long-Term Safety of HP and Other Immunization Methods) conditions diagnosed by a general practitioner (GP) are listed along the left. The treatment methods employed are listed with their measurements to show the odds ratio of the occurrence of these conditions. Methods assessed are HP only, conventional Vaccination, General homeopathic and other care only, or no intervention at all. There is an inverse relationship between the use of homeoprophylaxis and the long-term incidence of asthma, eczema, allergies and behavioral problems.

Chi Test P stands for what is known in statistics as the p-value. The p-value is a method of determining probability of the statistic found, or how likely it is that the observation occurred by chance (so the smaller the p-value the more reliable the statistic). The most significant p-values are bolded in the chart.

To quote Dr. Golden for his opinion regarding these findings, *"The explanation of this result remains open, but I would suggest that HP remedies stimulate the energetic immune response and this must lead to a maturing of the response in an analogous way that infection with simple diseases can help to mature the physical immune response."* [182]

In other words, triggering an immune response at the energetic level, using vibrational remedies as opposed to material doses of disease antigen, plays a role in maturing the immune system. This is accomplished in a way that is similar to how Mother Nature operates in the developing immune system – gently and carefully, single disease by single disease. [183]

---

[182] Golden, Isaac (2012). The Complete Practitioner's Manual of Homeoprophylaxis. Victoria, Australia. p 93.

[183] Golden, Isaac (2012). The Complete Practitioner's Manual of Homeoprophylaxis. Victoria, Australia. p 92.

Long-Term Safety of HP and Other Immunization Methods[184]

Condition: GP Diagnoses	Measurement	Method			
		HP-	Vaccin-	General	Nothing
Asthma	Odds	**0.124**	**1.89**	0.49	**0.69**
	Chi Test	**0.0006**	**0.0007**	0.13	6.5E-40
Eczema	Odds	**0.239**	**1.76**	0.225	0.665
	Chi Test	**0.0097**	**0.006**	**0.025**	6.5E-40
Ear/Hearing	Odds	0.703	**1.517**	0.599	**0.401**
	Chi Test	0.364	**0.04**	0.282	9.4E-41
Allergies	Odds	**0.307**	1.518	0.446	**0.608**
	Chi Test	**0.038**	0.061	0.171	5.8E-40
Behaviour	Odds	**0.541**	0.784	**1.675**	0.784
	Chi Test	**0.055**	0.613	**0.049**	1.2E-40

In his publication, The Complete Practitioner's Manual of Homeoprophylaxis," Dr. Golden states which results *"represent the first statistical evidence that long term homeoprophylaxis program may be associated with improvement of general health, as measured by a lower incidence of asthma, eczema, allergies and behavioral problems compared to vaccinated or unprotected children."* [185]

---

[184] Golden, Isaac (2012). The Complete Practitioner's Manual of Homeoprophylaxis. Victoria, Australia. p 92

[185] Golden, Isaac (2012). The Complete Practitioner's Manual of Homeoprophylaxis. Victoria, Australia. p 93.

Dr. Golden's early training in both statistics and economics impressed upon him the need for objective, data-based research in the area of homeoprophylaxis. Generations will benefit from his motivation to do so. His doctoral research at Swinburne University in Melbourne, Australia (2000-2004) focused upon evaluating the homeoprophylaxis program that provided nosodes for the childhood diseases typically covered by recommended vaccination programs.

A sample program will be illustrated in Chapter 11 providing the reader with the nuts and bolts of implementing homeoprophylaxis for your child.

In general, his research since 1985 has led him to conclude that while vaccination does provide a variable level of protection against many infectious diseases, its safety is not confirmed with any degree of certainty. In particular, long term health consequences of vaccines have not been adequately researched.

In comparison, homeoprophylaxis has provided 200 years of clinical evidence showing us that it is safe, devoid of any toxic components, and also yields positive long term health effects. [186] **And homeoprophylaxis appears from evidence to provide a level of protection which is comparable to or better than vaccines, meaning that parents have genuine choices available when it comes to preventing potentially serious infectious diseases.**

---

[186] Golden, Isaac (2012). The Complete Practitioner's Manual of Homeoprophylaxis. Victoria, Australia. p 118.

9 MAKING CHOICES

Every day I hear concern from parents about the choice to comply with the recommended vaccine schedule for babies and children. As mentioned earlier, in 2014, there are 39 recommended doses of diseases between birth and the first birthday. By the age of eighteen, over sixty-nine doses of diseases are being recommended. Young parents struggle to understand why these diseases are seen as such a threat when a generation ago most children had measles, mumps and chickenpox and survived to tell about it. Many young mothers in my own practice express surprise to hear that I only received four vaccines during my entire childhood.

Other moms, in an attempt to reduce the number of shots given to their babies are lulled into false complacency by being told that "this one shot will be all they need." In actuality, "this one shot" contains up to 5 combined diseases in some vaccines. One such vaccine contains diphtheria, tetanus, pertussin, hepatitis B and polio all in one injection. Another well-known vaccine contains diphtheria, tetanus, pertussin, HiB and polio.

The pediatrician says these are all necessary. There are multiple documents to sign if any of the vaccines are declined, informing you of what your decision could portend. The risks and responsibilities are spelled out in strong language. Here we have all the "authorities" saying there really is no choice if you are a responsible parent.

If you decline and navigate the legal exemption requirements, there's always some Aunt Harriet, or a mother-in-law bearing down on the topic with well-intended warnings. Fear of disease is a powerful motivator. Parents are especially vulnerable to this fear and worry. I remember as a first-time mother feeling the sobering immensity of responsibility for the life of this tiny, innocent being. What if I made a mistake? And it always felt as if there was also a long line of people behind me also thinking, "What if she makes a mistake?"

But who picks up the pieces if the doctor or vaccine manufacturer makes a mistake? Are they responsible for any injury incurred upon your child?

No. The responsibility is yours.

Responsibility

In 2005 the Public Readiness and Emergency Preparedness (PREPA) Act was passed by Congress. Vaccine manufacturers lobbied for this bill because it would preempt state vaccine safety laws in the case of an emergency declaration by Health and Human Services (HHS). In other words, state sanctioned vaccine exemptions would be null and void in the event of an emergency. This would apply to any vaccines rolled out for diseases such as anthrax, smallpox, H1N1, Ebola, or any perceived biological threat to citizens of the United States.

Furthermore, this blanket protection to vaccine manufacturers states that in order to file any legal claims for damages, one would have to prove "willful intention." In other words, proof that they intentionally brought to bear some degree of harm. This could not be tried in a public court of law, but only in a Health and Human Services court. The decision would be up to a physician employed by HHS. Maximum payment awards could not exceed $300,000. No duplicate insurance payments would be allowed, nor any payout whatsoever for legal fees, pain or suffering. [187]

PREPA combined with the Emergency Use Act (EUA), which allows the use of unlicensed vaccines [188] in an emergency, effectively removes all

---

[187] US Department of Health and Human Services. 2014. "PREP Act Q&As" Retrieved from:
http://www.phe.gov/Preparedness/legal/prepact/Pages/prepqa.aspx.

responsibility from vaccine manufacturers, public officials, clinics, medical doctors, and distributors of vaccines or anyone involved in the handling, distribution or sale of vaccines. In other words, the parent is fully and solely responsible.

So if you are made to feel "irresponsible" in the pediatrician's office, just remember that it is you who is the most responsible in the end.

The only way you can feel comfortable with the choices you make for your children is by getting all the information available to you. Then, with the information and freedom to choose, why would you make anything *but* **the best choice possible in any given situation? No one loves your child like you do. No one knows your child as well as you do. No one is on duty twenty four hours a day, 365 days a year for the care and nurturing of your child as you are. You are the expert.**

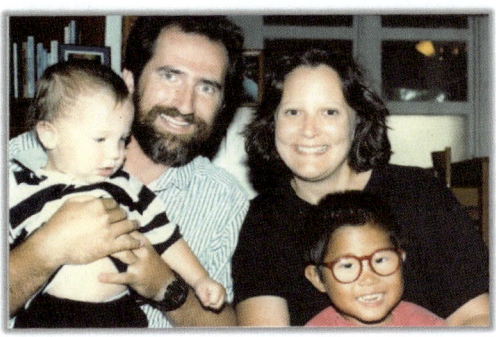

The value of having a good pediatrician is for support and additional information. Most pediatricians do not have time to do extensive research regarding vaccine science. Their days are filled with brief appointment slots governed by insurance company parameters and electronic medical record keeping. Immunizations are the only preventative medicine they have been taught to apply to their patients. Insurance company requirements dictate a "standard of care" that includes adherence to the recommended schedule of vaccines. Pediatricians risk being penalized for not complying.

You may have to look elsewhere for reliable information regarding vaccine safety. While alternative health care providers are frequently not covered

---

[188] U.S. Food and Drug Administration. "Emergency Use Authorizations Questions and Answers" webpage. Retrieved from: www.fda.gov/NewsEvents/PublicHealthFocus/ucm153297.htm.

under traditional health insurance policies, they are the ones who will spend more time with you and aim to individualize your health care. They may also be able to provide valuable insight about immunization due to their own study of the available research.

What about My Husband? Or Wife? Or Partner?

When a partner is reluctant to seek more information about vaccines, or has a preconceived bias, it can create much conflict. I've seen families torn apart by these differences. Each parent believes he/she knows best and is genuinely trying to convince the other. It can amount to a stalemate.

Resistance perpetuates resistance. Think of it this way: The very energy of resisting another's opinion causes that person to dig in harder in an effort to "convince." It's like one of those Chinese finger puzzles. You put a finger in each end and the harder you pull, the tighter it gets. Until you relax your hands, it's impossible to remove your fingers from the puzzle.

People sometimes come to me with a partner in hope that I will convince them of the risks of vaccines or the efficacy of homeoprophylaxis. My role in this situation is to listen and understand. When someone is truly "heard" they feel validated. Once they feel validated, they are actually able to listen without getting defensive. Once they realize that I have nothing to prove, they can consider listening a bit. All I want to do is empower parents. I've spent many years gathering information and seeing the clinical results of my patients. If I can share that with you, or your partner, you will have more information to make a good decision for your child.

How to Choose

There are some essential components to good choice making. The first goal is simply to **identify your goal.** What is your real motivation? Is it disease protection? Being a conscientious member of society? Respecting your pediatrician, or mother, or your college professor? Identify what is motivating you to choose one way or another. I've encountered parents whose chief motivation is to be "right" or to do something because that's what's always been done. Get clear about what's driving your choice.

Be teachable. Life is one big learning curve. We never know it all. And that's a good thing. The more we learn, the more we realize there is to learn. We continue to expand and grow and enlarge as a result of our experiences. Mistakes are part of the deal. If you think you will never make a mistake while raising your children, think again. They will surely remind you of all your mistakes when they hit their teen years! And I'm sure you can list some of the mistakes your own parents made. There is no such thing as perfect parenting. So admit you don't know it all and be teachable.

Be aware of biases. This can also be translated into "follow the money." Does the individual or organization have something to gain in the equation? Are they pressuring you in any way? Are they acting out of dogma or compulsion due to their own prejudices or because they are being influenced by someone or something to which they must comply? You can sense this if you have an uncomfortable feeling or feel pressured to make a decision immediately. This leads to the next important component of decision making.

Take your time. Life isn't a race. There are no deadlines. Maybe there are for paying your taxes, but raising your children is a lifelong journey. Give yourself permission to think about the choice you want to make. Try it on for size. Sleep on it. Allow yourself the time and space to feel good about how you want to proceed.

And lastly, follow your gut. Your instincts are good – especially when it comes to your children. You know the old saying, "Mothers have eyes in the back of their heads?" Well it's true. And so do dads. There are some things parents just "know" and this is intuition speaking. Intuition is a form of awareness and our awareness as human beings is expanding. It is wise to follow both your head and your heart in important matters. Weigh out the facts and listen to your intuition as well.

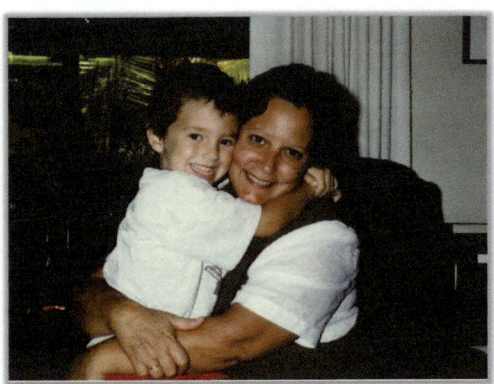

My goal is to empower parents. I want parents to feel the kind of support I wish I had when my children were small. I went from professional to specialist to expert over the years looking for answers. The advice they gave me often didn't work. It wasn't until I realized that I knew my children far better than they did that things started to change. Perhaps they had the education, but I was the mother and that 24/7 title qualified me to advocate for my children on their behalf. All I needed to do the best job was accurate information, authentic support and a little direction.

Your children and the decisions you must make on their behalf will cause you to grow beyond anything you imagined. You'll feel motivated to learn and understand topics you never thought you'd ever have any reason to explore. It's amazing how parenthood stretches us.

Often it's that which we lack that we try the hardest to find. And in that process of searching, we find that we have become enlarged, expanded. We have become more than we ever imagined ourselves to be. There's a gift of knowledge and experience in the place where we felt so inadequate. It's our weaknesses that make us strong. This is what happens as you struggle to make good choices for your children.

10 YOUR LEGAL RIGHTS

The first question many parents ask after deciding to use homeoprophylaxis is, can my child attend school without vaccines?

Three Exemptions

Each state in the U.S. has its own vaccine exemption laws. In 2014 all fifty states allow a medical exemption from vaccination. Forty-eight states allow an additional religious exemption and seventeen states have a third philosophical exemption.

The medical exemption must be signed by a medical doctor and is allowed for the following reasons:

- The child's immune status is compromised by a permanent or temporary condition. For example, the child might have a congenital condition leading to an impaired immune system. Or, the child might take medications, such as chemotherapy or steroids, which impair the immune system. In either case, vaccination could be harmful to the child's health.
- The child has a serious allergic reaction to a vaccine component.
- The child has had a prior serious adverse event related to vaccination. [189]

---

[189] The History of Vaccines. 2014 Retrieved from:

The two states allowing only a medical exemption are Mississippi and West Virginia.

Philosophical exemptions are easy to claim. They are also called "personal belief exemptions." You are required to fill out a form, either once or annually, for the public school district. This states that you are not vaccinating due to personal beliefs. See the map below for your state.

The state of Washington passed a law in 2011 requiring parents claiming personal belief exemptions must meet with a health care provider to discuss the risks and benefits of vaccination first.

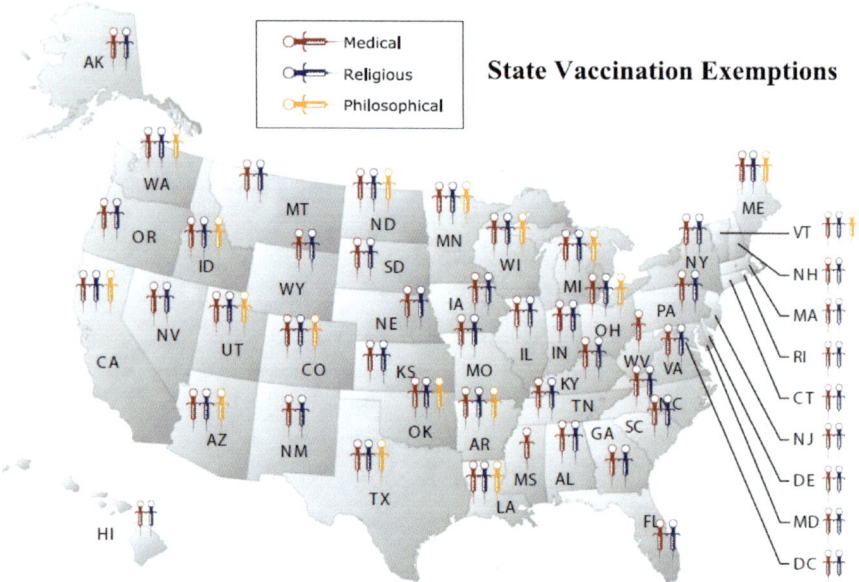

*As of June 2015, California joined West Virginia and Mississippi in removing religious and philosophical exemptions.[190]

This essentially makes it a bit more difficult to claim a philosophical exemption – requiring parents to jump through one more hoop. The stated intention is to provide accurate information before one chooses to decline vaccines.

---

http://www.historyofvaccines.org/content/articles/vaccination-exemptions

[190] 2014 Retrieved from:
http://www.generationrescue.org/resources/vaccination/exemption-laws-by-state-2/

Religious exemption can be viewed differently depending on which state you reside, which school district you are asking and who is sitting at the desk on the day you ask the question. For this reason, it's wise to understand the definition of religion made by the US Supreme Court. The Supreme Court states, Religion need not "be founded upon a belief in the fundamental premise of a 'God' as commonly understood in Western Theology."[191] The Court also states that, "the test of belief 'in relation to a Supreme Being' is whether a given belief that is sincere and meaningful occupies a place in the life of its possessor parallel to that filled by the orthodox belief in God."[192] Constitutionally, your rights allow you to claim a religious exemption simply because it is your sincerely held belief. It is not necessary to belong to an established religion.

While this sounds easy to claim a religious exemption, it can pose a slippery slope in some states. For this reason, I would advise you to contact Alan Phillips, JD, the only attorney in the United States who specializes in vaccine exemptions.

Alan can be reached through his website: www.vaccinerights.com

College Students and Health Care Employees

I receive numerous calls from parents of college students who are being asked to receive multiple vaccines in order to either attend classes, or fulfill clinical requirements while studying in the healthcare field. Public schools such as state colleges may qualify under state laws for exemptions. Other institutions may qualify under the 1964 Civil Rights Act as employers must allow appropriate accommodations for employees' religious beliefs.

Hospital employees are also often "required "to get the Hepatitis B vaccine.[193] According to Alan Phillips, this is not usually a formal requirement, but a recommendation by OSHA, a federal agency. He states, "As a federal agency, OSHA lacks authority to require immunizations of state residents." [194] There is an opt-out form that employees can sign to refuse the Hepatitis B vaccine. But it may still be possible for hospitals to require the Hepatitis B vaccine as a matter of company policy, even if OSHA only recommends it. [195]

---

[191] Sherr v. Northport-East Northport U. Free, 672 F. Supp. 81, 98 (E.D.N.Y. 1987) (quoting Torcaso v. Watkins, 367 U.S. 488, 81 S.Ct. 1680, 6 L.Ed.2d 982 (1961))
[192] Ibid

The latest trend in a number of public institutions such as nursing homes, hospitals and most recently, day care centers, has been to "require" employees to receive an annual influenza vaccination. If one declines, they are then required to wear a surgical mask throughout flu season, supposedly to protect others from their "unprotected" exhalations.

The Center for Disease Control does not support this notion. Their statement is as follows:

> "No recommendation can be made at this time for mask use in the community by asymptomatic persons, including those at high risk for complications, to prevent exposure to influenza. If unvaccinated high-risk persons decide to wear masks during periods of increased respiratory illness activity in the community, it is likely they will need to wear them any time they are in a public place and when they are around other household members."
>
> "However, no studies have definitively shown that mask use by either infectious patients or health-care personnel prevents influenza transmission." [196]

Furthermore, the Government Accountability Office notes that a program established a generation ago to help children injured by vaccines is now dominated by claims filed by adults who received a flu shot. Those cases typically claim that the adult suffered from Guillain-Barre Syndrome, in which the immune system attacks the nerves. [197]

---

[193] Phillips, A. (2013) The Authoritative Guide to Vaccine Legal Exemptions. Page 65.

[194] Ibid

[195] Ibid

[196] Centers for Disease Control and Prevention. Retrieved 2014 from: http://www.cdc.gov/flu/professionals/infectioncontrol/maskguidance.htm

[197] U.S. News and World Report Magazine. Retrieved 2014 from: http://www.usnews.com/news/us/articles/2014/11/21/feds-vows-to-publicize-vaccine-injury-help-%20program

And, more than 93,000 reports of reactions, hospitalizations, injuries and deaths following influenza vaccinations made to the federal Vaccine Adverse Events Reporting System (VAERS), including 1,080 related deaths, 8,888 hospitalizations, 1,801 related disabilities and over 1,700 cases of GBS. In 2013 the Federal Advisory Commission on Childhood Vaccines (ACCV) voted to add GBS to the Vaccine Injury Table within the federal Vaccine Injury Compensation Program (VICP). [198]

Travel Prophylaxis

Diseases that are endemic in a region can easily be included in a homeoprophylaxis program if one is traveling to an area where that disease is prevalent. Hepatitis, for instance, is one such disease. Dengue fever, typhoid, malaria, hepatitis A and others can also be included in a travel HP Program.

Many healthcare facilities are misinformed and will tell patients they must be vaccinated before traveling outside the United States. There are no legal requirements for vaccines when traveling other than the yellow fever vaccine for people traveling to and from some countries in sub-Saharan Africa and tropical South America where yellow fever is endemic.

Of course there are some common sense recommendations when traveling internationally. These include not drinking tap water, exercising caution when eating water-dense vegetables such as lettuce, and using bottled water to brush your teeth. In areas where there are mosquito-borne illnesses, consider mosquito netting if not staying in an air-conditioned hotel. Wearing long sleeves and pants will also reduce your exposure as a mosquito target.

When seeking homeoprophylaxis for travel, I always advise people to have an initial appointment a few months before intended travel. This allows time to determine which nosodes are needed and to get them mailed to you, allowing plenty of time to take them before you depart.

---

[198] National Vaccine Information Center. Retrieved 2014 from: http://www.nvic.org/vaccines-and-diseases/Influenza.aspx

Travel homeoprophylaxis needs to be assessed individually. Your actual plan will depend upon answers to questions such as, how long will you be there? Are you camping in the bush or staying in a four star hotel? Is your visit during the windy season (no mosquitoes) or the rainy season (lots of mosquitoes)?

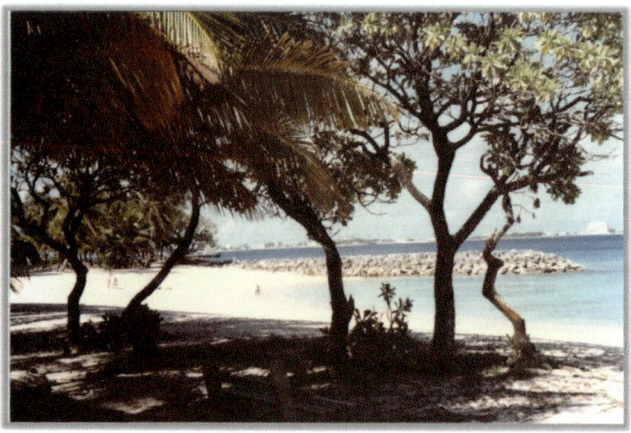

Within a brief consult we can usually determine exactly what your needs are for the trip and then provide the adequate nosodes.

You may consider repetition of nosode dosing for future travel depending on the length of time between trips. It's best to consult with your homeopath for exact direction.

11 APPLYING HOMEOPROPHYLAXIS

Once you've made the decision to use homeoprophylaxis, it's essential to locate a practitioner who can adequately support you. This means one who is able to provide you with the necessary remedies, is familiar enough with homeoprophylaxis to answer your questions, and also has some clinical experience in order to support you along the way as questions arise.

Dr. Golden has been providing his patients with a program since 1985 in Australia. Ravi Roy and Carola Lage-Roy have been offering an HP program for over forty years in Germany. Richard Hiltner, MD in California began using a form of homeoprophylaxis in the 1980's and even succeeded in having the state medical board approve his use of the standard vaccination record with "Homeoprophylaxis" stamped across the top.

Free and Healthy Children International (FHCI), the non-profit (501c3) organization I co-founded in 2012, identifies its mission as "providing education about HP and also training and supporting practitioners to administer HP." [199] FHCI also facilitated the collection of data from over 600 children using the program. This will be a valuable method to support Isaac Golden's findings of effectiveness and long-term health outcomes.

There are also many individual practitioners – homeopaths, naturopaths, or chiropractors who may be experienced and capable of supervising your family in a homeoprophylaxis program. Be sure to inquire if your particular practitioner is familiar with and practices homeoprophylaxis first.

The Plan

Most HP plans consist of regular doses of disease nosodes over an extended period of time. The value of spreading out the dosing over months and years is for optimum exposure to the vibrational influence of the remedies during maturation of the immune system.

The plan typically begins with a single dose of a relatively high potency of the nosode, such as a 200c. One month later, a triple dose of the same disease nosode, in the same potency, is given. The triple dose comprises three doses spread over a period of about twenty-four hours. They can be administered morning, noon and evening, or morning, night and next morning. Timing is not critical since this simply serves as an energetic reminder and need only be repeated three times within a period of approximately twenty-four hours.

The initial single dose "primes" the system. It alerts the vital force to the vibrational frequency of the disease in a gentle manner. The following triple dose a month later penetrates deeper into the system, carrying the message of the disease frequency. This is somewhat akin to providing the "software" to the system for the purpose of recognizing the actual disease if and when it is encountered in nature.

The following month the next disease is administered in the 200c potency for one single dose. One month after that, the same disease is given again three separate times within a twenty four hour period. This method is continued with each disease in turn. If a total of eight diseases are offered in an HP program, this dosing method would take approximately sixteen months to carry out. This segment of dosing is called "series one."

Once all the chosen diseases have been administered in 200c nosode form, the first disease on the list is revisited and administered in a 10M potency.

[199] www.freeandhealthychildren.com

This new potency is given in three separate doses within a twenty-four hour period. Now an even deeper resonance is attained within the system. Once all eight diseases have been given in triple doses of 10M potency, once per month, another eight months have elapsed. These doses of 10M potency are called "series two."

"Series three" consists of the same dosing protocol as series two. Once a month, three separate doses of 10m potency are given in a twenty-four hour period of each of the eight diseases in order. After this series, approximately thirty-two months have passed. I say "approximately" because there can be occasions when more or less than a month will pass between doses. More will be shared about this in the section entitled **Timing**.

The Pellets

A "dose" equals a few pellets. With homeopathy, it's never critical exactly how many pellets you give since it's energetic. Most people are so accustomed to conventional medicine and the risk of overdosing that parents always want to be certain of how many pellets are enough or too many. I usually tell them 2-4 pellets will be fine.

Do not touch the pellets with your bare hands. Oils from your hands may affect the pellets, so it's best to tap a few into the cap of the vial and then pour them into your child's mouth. Most children love taking the remedies as they are impregnated onto sugar pellets and melt easily.

With very young infants, it's possible to dissolve the pellets in a teaspoon of water and use a dropper or spoon to give a tiny dose. Again, the actual amount is not crucial. Getting any amount of water into the child's mouth is sufficient. Alternately, it's possible to place a pellet or two between the cheek and gum of a small infant and it will stick to the mucosa and melt. I have never had a baby choke on pellets as they stick readily and melt easily.

Remember to store your HP kit in a place where the temperature will not exceed 120 F, or 48 C. It is also best not to store remedies near strong smelling materials such as essential oils, Vicks Vapo-Rub, BenGay, Tiger Balm or Eucalyptus. These strong scents can deactivate the remedies. Other risky storage areas would include near a microwave, television, or computer. It's also best not to expose your remedies to bright sunlight. If you observe these simple measures, homeopathic remedies will last indefinitely. They never expire. If you see an "expiration date" on the vial, don't be confused. They are made in FDA approved homeopathic pharmacies and the FDA requires an expiration date on each vial.

An interesting fact is that the physician and senator, Royal S. Copeland, MD, was a practicing homeopath and primary author and sponsor of the Federal Food, Drug and Cosmetic Act of 1938. He was responsible for including the Homeopathic Pharmacopoeia of the United States (HPUS) to assure that homeopathic medications are safe, accessible and legal in the United States.[200]

Timing

The one month dosing schedule is completely flexible. It can be shortened to as close as every two weeks or doses can be spaced much farther apart than four weeks due to illness, vacation schedules or memory loss!

The younger the infant the more closely you should adhere to the one month dosing schedule. This respects their developing immune system and provides the energetic influence of the diseases over a longer period of time. Under the age of two they are at more risk for diseases such as pertussis, so rushing through the dosing isn't recommended.

For example: If the program is started at one month of age, they would receive a single 200c dose of pertussis at one month, a triple dose of 200c at two months, then a triple dose of 10M at seventeen months and again at twenty-five months. This provides continuous 'information' about the disease communicated to the child's vital force over the period of two years.

Dr. Golden has speculated that immunity may last for at least ten years after the completion of this schedule, provided the patient is not exposed to severe shocks or traumas which can imbalance the immune system. After that time, boosting doses of homeoprophylaxis may be administered if desired. [201]

Since it is never advisable to give the HP dose when a child is sick, it is possible that periods longer than one month may elapse between doses. Some of my patients in Minnesota, where temperatures stay in the single digits for months at a time in the winter, may have multiple months go by

---

[200] American Association of Homeopathic Pharmacists. 2014 Retrieved from: http://www.aahp.info/regulatory/overview-of-homeopathic-drug-product-regulation/

[201] Golden, Isaac. 2014. Toronto Canada Lecture "Homeoprophylaxis."

between doses. If all the children in a family are on HP and happen to be passing around a virus, it's sometimes easier to have everyone on the same schedule, so Mom will wait until everyone is well. There have been cases where it takes until the spring thaw to resume dosing.

The opposite example of shortening the time between doses would be completely acceptable for a child over the age of two. If a family trip is coming up you may want to administer a dose before traveling, so you don't have to pack and carry along the kit. If a particular disease is showing up in the neighborhood and you want to be sure and have your child familiar with that nosode, by all means, shorten the schedule and proceed with the dose.

If your child is sick, always wait at least forty-eight hours after he or she is completely well to administer the next dose. Remember that the immune system can effectively manage one disease at a time. Allow time for either the naturally occurring disease process or the energetic disease in the form of a nosode to be recognized and responded to adequately.

This wonderful flexibility makes the HP program completely adaptable to families and individuals. Moreover, the process of observing your child in this way deepens your understanding of how his immune system is functioning. The knowledge that one disease at a time is being navigated by your child's developing immunity gives you a different perspective than the fear of disease promulgated by a medical community that erroneously believes wellness is simply the absence of symptoms.

Which Diseases

Young mothers today have been unduly influenced by emphasis on the fear of disease. Along the street, every five hundred yards there's a sign advertising flu vaccines. Grocery stores, drugstores and work places have "specials" on the annual flu shot. Elementary schools are providing them on site with the casualness of passing out cartons of milk. This is truly a marketing marvel.

How many deaths actually occur as a result of the flu? The American Journal of Epidemiology published a study assessing mortality from the flu in the United States, over a period of twenty-two years (from 1979 to 2001). The total number of deaths during that period were 41,400. This number divided by twenty-two years amounts to 1881 deaths per year. [202] Many of these deaths were from the development of pneumonia, which homeopaths know can occur when fever is suppressed in the body's effort to resolve influenza.

Influenza is not a deadly disease to be feared. If desired, the nosode called influenzinum can be taken yearly for the annual flu circulating. It's important to take a look at just which diseases we need protection from and which diseases we do not.

What I include in my own program is similar to Dr. Golden's original program. They are:

- Pertussis (whooping cough)
- Pneumonia
- Haemophilus B
- Polio
- Meningitis
- Mumps
- Measles
- Tetanus

These are the diseases which have either existed in epidemic proportions historically, or have significant mortality rates. They are not the multiple viruses that circulate providing mild and beneficial exposure to the developing immune systems of children.

Let's discuss those diseases *not* included in the HP program.

The shift towards pre-emptive strikes on disease first occurred with the advent of the hepatitis B vaccine. At an incidence of less than 1% in the United States, hepatitis B is hardly an epidemic, yet this vaccine was added to the recommended list in 1991. It was recommended for infants beginning at twelve hours old, with two subsequent doses by the age of eighteen months. [203]

---

[202] American Journal of Epidemiology. Dushoff, J, Plotkin, J, et al. Mortality due to Influenza in the United States—An Annualized Regression Approach Using Multiple-Cause Mortality Data.2005 Retrieved 2014 from: http://aje.oxfordjournals.org/content/163/2/181.full

[203] National Vaccine Information Center. 2014 Retrieved from: http://www.nvic.org/vaccines-and-diseases/Hepatitis-B.aspx

So when parents ask why hepatitis B isn't on the homeoprophylaxis schedule of diseases, I first ask them if they feel their infant is at risk for a sexually transmitted disease. If not, and they plan to be traveling to a country where hepatitis B is prevalent later in life, they can always add that nosode to the schedule. Realistically speaking, Hep B is given in the hospital at birth in order to get parents compliant to a schedule of continued immunizations.

Diphtheria is not included as there have been only two cases in the United States recorded in the 21st century.[204] There has been some resurgence in India, so those living or traveling there may want to consider this nosode.[205] If it's of any concern, it can easily be added to the schedule.

Chickenpox was addressed in Chapter 2, The Big Business of Vaccines, with its risk of increasing cases of shingles. Interestingly, in 2006 the CDC recommended an additional booster shot of chickenpox vaccine for all children. That was the same year a shingles vaccine was licensed and recommended for all adults over age 60. It's interesting to note that the efficacy of this vaccine is only 44%. Additionally, the varicella vaccine was one of the first to be grown on human diploid cell cultures, thus increasing rates of immune disorders amongst children.

By not including chickenpox in the HP program, many parents are still seeking wild cases, so they can expose their children for a healthy dose of the real disease. It is available in nosode form and can be added to the program at any time.

Rotovirus is not included since it was discussed in Chapter 4, Vaccine Studies. If you are living in an undeveloped nation with difficult access to clean water, you may want to consider adding this nosode to the program. Or rotovirus can be treated very effectively with other homeopathic remedies once contracted.

Prevnar is a vaccine designed to prevent common strains of pneumococcal bacteria. It was banned in Holland in 2009 after three infant deaths within a two week period. [206] It was also banned in Japan in 2011 after the deaths

---

[204] Centers for Disease Control and Prevention. 2014 retrieved from: http://www.cdc.gov/mmwr/preview/mmwrhtml/mm6311md.htm#tab1

[205] Indian J Med Res 128, November 2008, pp 669-670 Retrieved 2014 from: http://medind.nic.in/iby/t08/i11/ibyt08i11p669.pdf

[206] Retrieved 2014 from: http://www.zentrum-der-

of four babies shortly after receiving it.[207] The HP nosode called pneumococcinum addresses immunity to pneumococcal bacteria.

Rubella is also not included but can be added when children reach childbearing age. While this is a relatively mild virus, if contracted during the first twelve weeks of pregnancy, it can result in severe birth defects such as deafness, mental retardation or cardiac abnormalities. [208] It makes sense to provide protection closer to the time a woman is likely to become pregnant.

Gardasil

Human Papillomavirus (HPV) is not included in an HP program. In 2009 I attended a seminar where Diane Harper, MD lectured. Dr. Harper is one of the leading authorities on HPV and was consulted by the pharmaceutical company Merck in the development of the Gardasil vaccine. Her information was eye-opening.

From Dr. Harper I learned that 60% of women who are sexually active naturally contract HPV. Of the 100-plus strains of HPV, only about thirteen of them are responsible for cervical cancer. Even the low risk strains can cause abnormal pap smears. While this can result in much anxiety for women, it is often unfounded. It takes five to thirty years for untreated HPV to develop to cancer, so it's very slow growing. Caught in time it is 100% treatable. [209]

Of those 60% of sexually active women infected with HPV, 90% of them will spontaneously clear the virus within two years with no treatment at all. If women are receiving annual pap smears, any changes will be detected very early. [210]

---

gesundheit.de/pdf/impfstoff-verbot-japan-ia_03.pdf

[207] Politicol News. Retrieved 2014 from: http://www.politicolnews.com/pfizer-prevnar-13-read-the-fine-print/

[208] The Mayo Clinic. 2014 retrieved from: http://www.mayoclinic.org/diseases-conditions/rubella/basics/complications/con-20020067

[209] Fourth International Conference on Vaccination. National Vaccine Information Center. October 2009.

[210] Ibid

She went on to say that efficacy in women younger than fifteen has not been established. 30% of those immunized lose antibodies in three years and actual duration of immunity is unknown. No data has been collected determining what happens if a woman is given the vaccine prior to becoming pregnant. No "herd immunity" is established with HPV vaccines. They do NOT protect against cervical cancer; they protect against two strains of HPV (16 and 18). Thirteen high risk strains cause 70% of cervical cancers.

And lastly she emphasized that efficacy can only be expected if the vaccine is given two years prior to beginning sexual activity, and yearly pap screening must still be done. Her personal commentary, in light of limited testing prior to marketing a vaccine for HPV, was that this was "one giant public health experiment." [211]

Here's the homeopathic perspective: We know that HPV is a naturally occurring virus that clears itself in the vast majority of cases. It is slow growing and 100% curable. Are we once again toying with nature in an attempt to change something that doesn't need to be changed? Are we repeating the varicella debacle and encouraging an increase of other pathology down the road?

Responses to Homeoprophylaxis Dosing

There are no "toxic reactions" to homeoprophylaxis. What you may see is an immune "response." This is a desired effect. The response may appear as a bit of fussiness, a missed nap, perhaps a low fever, or even a flushed face or temporary rash. If you are questioning a response, you should always contact your practitioner. It is impossible to acquire an infectious disease from homeoprophylaxis remedies.

One of the first questions your practitioner will ask is, "What is your child doing? Is he or she playing, eating, drinking, urinating?" If so, then we can conclude that their vitally is good. A child can have a 102 F. (38 C.) degree fever and still have good vitality if we observe few or no limiting symptoms. We define this as a healing fever. A healing fever is the body's response to an illness that illustrates the innate curative power of a child's robust immune system. This is a good thing.

---

[211] Ibid

Typically this will pass relatively soon. I've had moms call me with a thermometer in hand, fretting over a 99 degree temperature and a flushed face. When I learn that the baby is eating, drinking and giggling at siblings, I reassure her that this is a good immune response. She should watch and let me know if it doesn't resolve within the next 12-24 hours.

Most mothers are amazed when the fever leaves as quickly as it arrived. They see a happy baby with no signs of distress. Welcome to homeoprophylaxis!

Part of the value of homeoprophylaxis is learning to observe your child in sickness and in health, in a way that helps you to understand what's happening physically, emotionally, and immunologically. When a child has a naturally occurring virus and is under the weather for a few days, we often see a surge of development once they are well. It's as if the system was using all its energy to mount a response to the illness and once that's accomplished, the momentum continues in a new developmental leap. I've seen children say their first words, master new skills, or blossom socially once better.

I have had mothers report that they see this phenomenon as well after giving doses of HP. The child is receiving the benefits of an energetic disease. There are no risks as there would be with the actual material disease. They received this energetic disease with pellets in the mouth, so initial immune responses could initiate in the mucous membrane. This is the natural order of things. There were no preservatives, adjuvents, detergents or antibiotics included, so the response could be unhindered by attempts to expel toxins. And they received one single disease, allowing the body to mount a response and complete the cycle naturally.

If your child is not 100% better from any immune response by the next day, your practitioner may advise you to give an additional dose of the nosode. In effect, this will provide a gentle bump to move forward. The immune response is a bit stuck and needs a reminder. I sometimes tell parents that it's like a car spinning its wheels in a snowbank. It just needs a bit of traction to move ahead.

A Natural Illness?

There is always a chance that your child contracted a natural illness just prior to taking the nosode. Healthy children *do* pick up multiple viruses each year; many going unnoticed except for very slight symptoms. In this event, the symptoms you see are not an immune response to the particular HP dose just given. Your practitioner will help you determine what is actually happening. Before long, you will be able to distinguish this as well.

In the event of a different illness, you have a choice to wait and see, or to have your practitioner assist you in treating it acutely. Once your child is well for 48 hours you would re-dose the nosode you just gave. Remember, the body addresses one illness at a time.

If your child is sick prior to a scheduled dose, wait. Make sure he or she is well for 48 hours before giving the scheduled nosode. Remember the schedule is completely flexible and waiting a bit longer is no problem.

Travel Prophylaxis

If you want to add any disease nosodes into your program, this is easy to do. Refer to the section in Chapter 10 about travel HP. Additionally, just let your practitioner know in plenty of time prior to travelling. The necessary nosodes can be included in the foundational homeoprophylaxis program. In fact, the entire family can easily take the travel nosodes.

What If My Child Is Vaccinated?

Some parents discover homeoprophylaxis after starting out using a conventional schedule of vaccination. Perhaps they had some concerns and used a modified plan. They wonder if they can also use HP and if so, what should they expect?

Homeoprophylaxis can be used with any child who is neuro-typical and immune-typical. Children who suffer from asthma, eczema, chronic upper respiratory infection, developmental delays, or other chronic conditions should be evaluated on an individual basis. Some of these children can be treated homeopathically, regain a new level of health and go on to use homeoprophylaxis to further educate their immune system.

If you believe your child suffered permanent ill effects from vaccination or other environmental influences, you may want to explore CEASE therapy. This is a method devised by Tinus Smits, MD and used to eliminate autism spectrum expression. Read more about this in Chapter 12.

If your child received some or all of the recommended vaccines, you do not suspect permanent vaccine damage, and you would like to pursue homeoprophylaxis, this is easily done. Perhaps you saw a response that worried you after a vaccine such as excessive shrill crying, or a change in behavior. Maybe you have done some research and don't feel comfortable with the vaccine ingredients or method of administration any longer.

These children can manifest a more pronounced immune response after taking HP nosodes for the following reason. A developing immune system confused by the repeated administration of eight or more diseases at one time is trying to reorder itself. The innate intelligence involved in mounting an immune response and following through to resolution has been confused. With repetition of a single disease (homeoprophylaxis) at a time, this can be relearned, or perhaps it's more accurate to say, remembered.

It's possible to observe an immune response that doesn't resolve until another dose of nosode is given, or perhaps a different homeopathic remedy. After practicing this exercise a few times, the immune system can start to recall how to function more normally, generating a mild immune response, resolving it and moving forward.

Long Term Health Outcomes

What will we see in these children five, ten, or twenty years from now? The answers to this question will continue to unfold as the work of people such as Isaac Golden, Gustavo Bracho, Francisco Eizayaga, and others moves forward. Individuals not financed by large pharmaceutical companies are working tirelessly, fueled by personal motivations, commitment to the art and science of healing, or perhaps personal dharma.

We know homeoprophylaxis is safe. No one has ever died or been permanently injured from using it. The same cannot be said about vaccines. Why is there no requirement to assure safety? If a stroller, or crib, or toy caused a child to be injured or die, it would be removed from the market immediately. Why is this not so with vaccines?

The rising epidemic of chronically ill children is a devastation, not only to the hearts and homes of loving parents, but also to our economy and future. If one in 10,000 children suffered from autism in the 1950's and one in 50 is on the autism spectrum in 2014, how many will be afflicted in the decade to come? Autism is just one of the severe chronic illnesses among children we see increasing exponentially. Asthma, auto-immune disorders, and neurological conditions are now commonplace, when they were once rarely seen in pediatric populations.

The father of immunology and Nobel Prize winner, Dr. Emil Adolf von Behring, discovered in 1901 that homeopathic remedies produced enhanced immunogenic activity. He was pressured by his colleagues to hide his initial results. He did so until he was awarded the Nobel Prize when he then made public his discovery. [212]

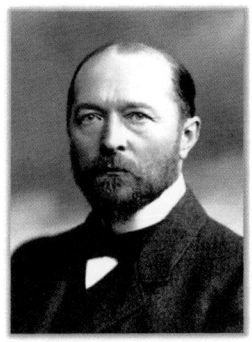

Dr. Emil Adolf von Behring

If we know something is safe after 200 years of use and we know that it produces improved immunological responses, it makes sense to think that we will see an improvement in health over time.

---

[212] Malik, N. Retrieved 2014 from: http://drnancymalik.wordpress.com/2012/06/05/nobel-prize-winners-on-homeopathy/

12 CEASE THERAPY

CEASE stands for "Complete Elimination of Autistic Spectrum Expression." It is a therapy devised by the late Tinus Smits, MD, a Dutch physician deeply touched by the suffering of children. His method has been successfully used by hundreds of practitioners throughout Europe, North and South America, as well as many Asian countries. Practitioners must be certified in the method and training seminars are taught in Europe, the United States, and throughout the world. [213]

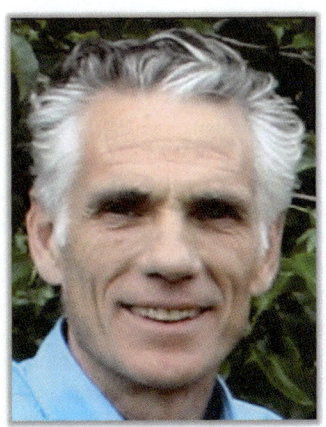

Dr. Tinus Smits

---

[213] 2014 retrieved from: www.cease-therapy.com

CEASE Therapy primarily addresses obstacles to cure. These might be obstacles of varying origin. Many have associated CEASE Therapy with the reversal of vaccine injury, but it can successfully remove obstacles such as environmental poisonings, chronic allergies or damage caused by allopathic medications. The method consists of three components that must be understood and utilized in relationship to each other in a balanced and dynamic way.

The components are: 1) orthomolecular therapy, 2) isotherapy and 3) the "Saturday Remedy," comprised of Inspiring Homeopathy, also known as IH, Classical Homeopathy, the use of sarcodes, bowel nosodes or other modalities. This last component the "Saturday Remedy," may shift and change as needed.

Orthomolecular Therapy

Many non-CEASE practitioners who specialize in treating children on the autism spectrum employ the use of multiple supplements. This can sometimes have a contradictory effect upon already taxed systems. It requires energy to assimilate supplements and autistic children who are loaded with many different medications can sometimes show improvement just by reducing supplementation to only the most essential components.

CEASE Therapy recommends just a few main supplements that are dynamically adjusted up or down in dosage based upon individual response from the child. Within the training, recommendations are made for the highest quality orthomolecular supplements based upon ongoing research. None of these are necessarily obtained through multilevel marketing (MLM) companies, and patients are free to choose the brands they wish.

Isotherapy

Isotherapy within the context of CEASE Therapy refers to the use of potentized homeopathic remedies made from the same substances suspected of causing damage. In many cases this is a vaccine, but not in every case. Different medications, anesthesia, or environmental exposures can all result in continued toxicity and ill effects. The administration of these isotherapeutic remedies result in the body's natural ability to detoxify. More will follow regarding detoxification as I explain how the three methods are employed.

Inspiring Homeopathy

Inspiring Homeopathy, or IH, was also devised by Dr. Smits. He postulated that individuals possess seven shared universal layers. These layers focus upon self-confidence, self-love, incarnation to a human body, protection and victimization, duality and connection with one's soul. Imbalances in these layers can be addressed with IH remedies. Nine commonly known homeopathic remedies made from animal, mineral and vegetable substances are given intermittently. These result in much needed support of individual evolution. As mentioned, IH remedies, classical homeopathic remedies or other specialized classes of remedies are chosen to be given once a week, as the "Saturday Remedy."

The Dynamic Balance

The art and science of applying CEASE Therapy depends upon careful observation of an individual's response and subsequent adjustment of the above three components. CEASE is not about applying a rigid protocol. It requires sensitivity, finesse and sharp clinical skills.

I have intentionally not included essential details of the three components required so that attempts are not made to try this on one's own. CEASE cannot be learned from a book, nor is it within the scope of this book to provide the necessary instruction. Please seek out a certified and experienced CEASE practitioner by visiting **www.cease-therapy.com**.

Parents seeking CEASE Therapy must also understand that this process engages the child's vital force in such a way as to elicit organic healing on a very deep level. It is not about treating symptoms alone. It is not an overnight, quick fix. Time and patience are requirements. I have seen some cases move very quickly in a matter of weeks or months, while others can take much longer to obtain the same progress.

Tinus said, "The birth of a child is a miracle. Keeping a child healthy is an art." It is this process of part miracle and part art that imbues the therapy with such success. Initially an in depth history is taken. Careful attention must be paid to when symptoms began along with every nuance of the child's emotional and physical constitution. The parent's information is also important. What was the mental state of each parent during the time of conception? Were any drugs taken regularly prior to conception or during pregnancy? What was the labor and delivery like? These questions and more will comprise the initial case taking session.

A thorough timeline can then be constructed identifying the chronological order of symptoms, complaints, behavioral changes, developmental milestones or delays. The practitioner constructs a plan, addressing what is asking to be addressed in the case. Perhaps this will begin with an IH remedy. Often it can begin with the simple addition of some orthomolecular supplements. At times, the isopathic remedy is loud and clear and provides the starting point. No two cases are alike. A single component must be evaluated individually. At each step along the way we can add or change a component, one at a time, slowly and carefully. The child is the guide.

If a specific pharmaceutical is identified as a culprit, that particular drug can be obtained in a homeopathic dilution to be used isopathically for "clearing" the obstacle in the way of healing. As each isopathic dose is given, careful evaluation determines where the child is in the process. At some point an IH remedy may be called for, or an increase or decrease of orthomolecular supplements. No two cases follow the same course. Each step along the way, open communication between parent and practitioner as well as astute observation will guide the course of treatment forward.

Following are two cases addressed with CEASE Therapy.

CEASE With a Young Adult

Beverly (not her actual name) came to me looking shaky and pale. She had not slept well for weeks and had been to multiple doctors seeking answers. No one could diagnose her and one by one sent her home with instructions to rest with a tone in their voice suggesting that perhaps this was just stress or anxiety. They of course tried all the usual tools of the trade – spinal taps to search for bizarre microbes lurking in her cerebrospinal fluid, blood work, urine analyses, and more to try and nail down a diagnosis. Then antibiotics, antifungals, steroids, as well as antidepressants to try to diagnose by elimination. Nothing worked. Her transient pain, stiff neck, sleeplessness, vomiting, anxiety and mouth full of blisters continued unabated.

Beverly was the child of chiropractors. She had never been vaccinated and at twenty years old was healthy and rarely ill as a child. Until now. What had changed?

Beverly was about to attend medical school. The prerequisite was to be fully vaccinated. So within a period of about two months, she received all of her vaccines. All of them! Measles, mumps, rubella, pertussis, tetanus, diphtheria, hepatitis A, hepatitis B, meningitis, and a flu shot for good measure. Almost immediately she began to decline. As doctors searched for a cause, vaccination was disregarded. Of course vaccinations are assumed safe.

Here was clear etiology and I set to work to distinguish which vaccine should be cleared first. I decided upon the tetanus vaccine and identified that she had received a commonly administered shot containing a tetanus, diphtheria and pertussis combination used for adults. It contains Polysorbate 80.

Polysorbate 80 has the ability to penetrate the blood brain barrier, delivering a fast track to the brain for any other chemical in the vaccine. Additionally, this particular vaccine is grown on a medium containing a bovine (cow) extract. [214] Interesting to note was that Beverly was a vegan.

Within one week of starting treatment, Beverly was beginning to improve. Her sleep became more regular, she could eat without vomiting and the blisters in her mouth began to heal. By week three of treatment she was improved by 80%. Her parents had no doubt that vaccines were the cause.

CEASE With an Infant

Troy (not his actual name) was a 'premie'. He was born about two weeks early and weighed barely five pounds. He was alert and healthy and his parents were proud and relieved. An enthusiastic young nurse, committed to fulfilling her responsibilities, gave Troy a hepatitis B immunization when he was less than 24 hours old. All seemed to progress well and Troy's parents took him home when he was chubby enough to be discharged. He was a good feeder, mom had an ample milk supply and he continued to thrive.

At two months Troy was taken into the pediatrician who gave him his first round of vaccinations. Hep B, polio, DTaP, and Rotovirus. Suddenly something was different. He no longer made eye contact during feedings. He fussed and cried excessively for no apparent reason, clenching his hands into tight little fists all the time. There was something about him that felt like "he was just not there" reported his mother during our intake appointment.

She had waited to bring him back in to the doctor until his four month well-baby checkup. She thought she might be imagining things. But the

[214] Centers for Disease Prevention and Control 2014 retrieved from: http://www.cdc.gov/vaccines/pubs/pinkbook/downloads/appendices/b/excipient-table-2.pdf

doctor confirmed that something wasn't quite right and decided to "hold off" on the second round of shots. He mentioned the word "autism" and this terrified his mom. She halted all vaccines at that time.

It was almost a year later when I finally met with Troy. Taking a careful case, I determined that the hepatitis B vaccine needed to be cleared. We started immediately and after his first dose Troy began to scream. Mom was amazed, saying, "This is how he sounded when he got his shots." He had a rough few hours of agitation and red-faced crying. We quickly introduced the correct orthomolecular supplements to ease the detoxing that was taking place.

Troy settled down and sailed through the following doses of the clearing remedy. Within a week he was back to his old self, making good eye contact, giggling and responding to mom and siblings in an appropriate way. His fists unclenched and he was back to being sweet baby Troy.

Note: no child under the age of a year should undertake detox unless under the experienced and watchful eye of a certified CEASE Therapist, licensed physician or naturopath.

These two cases were wonderfully clear to evaluate and treat. In following up, both these patients went on to have no further symptoms and continued to thrive. Not every case is as straight forward or as quickly responsive. Some are more challenging to understand from the beginning. Some are layered with many different offending agents that must be carefully unpeeled and balanced with supplemental support, IH remedies and homeopathic remedies, and support of the parents with tender patience and perseverance.

CEASE Therapy is not required in every case. There are other cases of children on the autism spectrum who respond beautifully to classical homeopathy and nutritional support. Parents should carefully do their research and locate a practitioner with whom they feel comfortable. Parents should not attempt to employ CEASE Therapy on their own.

Healing is a lifelong process that requires planning and execution. The healthy child is the child who is adaptable – able to get sick and get better. Unlike advertising would have us believe, health is not a destination to which we arrive and remain, never to be sick again. And Titus reminds us, "Keeping a child healthy is an art."

13 CONCLUSION

As a child, my dreams were simple. I wanted to be a mother. I fantasized about having a large family of adorable children, glowing and obedient. They would be loving and happy and healthy. I would bake them bread, braid their hair and bandage their hurts. My simple dream turned out to be not so simple after all.

Navigating infertility and then adoption was confusing, overwhelming and more challenging than I ever envisioned. Once I had children, questions and problems arose that seemed insurmountable. I realized that sleeping, eating and eliminating are three functions that cannot be controlled in another human being. I couldn't make everything right.

A tiny infant can be so helpless, yet so powerful. My life was continuously adapting around the needs of these mysterious creatures. Motherhood was nothing like I imagined. What happened to all my perfect plans? My children elicited emotions I never even knew existed! Exhaustion magnified every emotion. There were days, perhaps even years, when I questioned what I had done. Why did I struggle so hard to have children when they brought so many insurmountable problems? Everywhere I turned there was another hurdle, or another decision to be made. Each decision felt so important, so potentially life changing. What if I ruined it all? What if my children grew up and never wanted to speak to me again?

No one raises perfect children. No one is exempt from making mistakes. The human condition is one of trial and error. We learn as we go. It stinks, but it's reality. Actually, it's the best way. Without the contrast of feeling miserable, we would never savor the deliciousness of life; nor strive to obtain a better condition. It's the struggle that motivates us to seek the calm. And the struggles inspire us to envision exactly what we *do* want in our lives. By envisioning what we want, we move towards it, consciously and subconsciously step by step.

My steps led me to where I am now. Was I a perfect mother? No. Far from it. But my children are still speaking to me. In fact, we have wonderful and rich relationships. I love the people they have become.

Your story will not unfold like mine. Be grateful for your own. Through it you will access the riches of learning who you are and who these people are who you call your children. Do your homework and find your own answers. Don't take my word for it.

You possess everything you need to be equal to the task. It's called love. It's a force that can shape lives and move mountains. It can jump in front of a speeding car, feed and nurture a tiny baby, or find a lost Lego piece to forestall a tantrum. No one can deliver it to your child in exactly the same way that you can. In this regard, you and I are not so different.

This book presents a challenge to the reader. Where do I go from here? My greatest hope is that you will access the references provided and do your own research. Become your own healer, armed with the light of your own studies and conclusions. Make the best decisions possible for the health of your children and family.

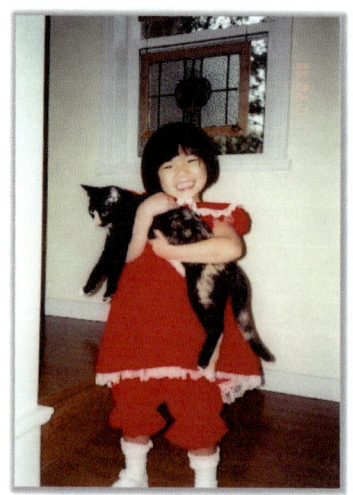

Lily with the cat

ABOUT THE AUTHOR

Cilla Whatcott grew up in Little Silver, New Jersey. She has lived on the east coast of the United States, on the west coast, aboard a sailboat off the coast of Florida, and ten years in the Republic of the Marshall Islands.

She attended Arizona State University where she graduated with a bachelor's degree in Dance and awarded the honor of "Most Outstanding Student." She choreographed, performed and taught dance in Arizona, the Republic of the Marshall Islands and Whidbey Island, Washington.

She and her husband, Neal, have adopted children from Taiwan, China and Russia and have one biological son, born to them in the beautiful Marshall Islands.

Cilla graduated from the four year professional program in homeopathic medicine at Northwestern Academy of Homeopathy in Minneapolis, Minnesota. In 2015 she earned her PhD in homeopathy from Kingdom College of Natural Health. In addition to a private healing practice, Cilla teaches classes in homeopathy at Normandale Community College in Bloomington, Minnesota, serves on the research faculty of The American Medical College of Homeopathy, is a mentor of students at Northwestern Academy of Homeopathy and Teleosis Homeopathic Collaborative, the co-founder of Free and Healthy Children International and co-author of *"The Solution: Homeoprophylaxis the Vaccine Alternative."*

Driven by equal parts curiosity and compassion, Cilla spends her days working with vaccine damaged children, mentoring student homeopaths and researching minutiae that make a difference. While she survived both the paperwork and challenges posed by parenting an international family, her deepest desire remains to be known as a good enough mother.

She can be reached at:
cilla.whatcott@gmail.com or **www.familyhomeopathycare.com**

SOME THANK YOUS

Each of us is the unfolding result of experiences, individuals and influences that touch our lives. While we often assume that thanks need be doled out to those who have provided the most love, support, and encouragement, I also believe that those who have posed the greatest difficulties and challenges have indeed been the greatest teachers and guides along the way. They deserve our gratitude. Understanding the larger picture may be required to feel true appreciation for those who have caused pain and consternation. The happy news is that once on the other side of this material life, they will probably be the ones to whom we run with open arms and thank for the resulting leaps in growth and understanding they facilitated. I will leave these individuals unnamed while I quietly thank them in my heart.

My public appreciation goes to many. I offer my apologies to any of you I have inadvertently left out. Thank you to Mr. Maloney – my 7th grade teacher who awarded me first prize in a writing contest and brought to my awareness that perhaps I liked to express myself in writing; David Saltman- for really listening; my family in New Jersey (Pat, Laverne and Patti) where despite the turnpike and oil refineries, it was an idyllic place to grow up; Niki, and Diane – you are synonymous with Kwajalein and the best time in my life; Kim – for your enormous spirit and constant encouragement; Helen – for your wild, free walk in both worlds at once; Tilak – for your wakeup call; MM and CL for your patience in showing me the way; Isaac – for your editing, your kindness and encouragement; Max- for your wonderful max-ness; Gus- for your heart and for keeping me on my toes; Lily- for your sweet mysterious independence; Inga – for your resilience and transformation; and to Neal – my best friend, my lifelong partner, my sounding board, handyman, emotional diffuser, counselor, co-analyzer, editor, illustrator and more. You have encouraged our unique international family, had endless patience with my shortcomings, always built wings beneath my creative ideas and have been the solid support enabling us to embrace it all. Living life with you makes me unbelievably happy.

Disclaimer: The information contained in this book is purely educational. It is not intended to replace the advice of your medical practitioner. The reader takes sole responsibility for any decisions made regarding health and wellbeing as a result of reading *There Is a Choice*.

Printed in Dunstable, United Kingdom